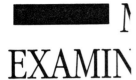 

EXAMINATION

OCCUPATIONAL
THERAPY

FIFTH EDITION

800
Multiple-Choice Questions with
Referenced, Explanatory Answers

H. DWYER DUNDON
M.A., O.T.R., F.A.O.T.A.
Associate Professor of Occupational Therapy
School of Health Related Professions
University of Missouri
Columbia, Missouri

MEDICAL EXAMINATION PUBLISHING COMPANY

Notice: The author(s) and the publisher of this volume have taken care that the information and recommendations contained herein are accurate and compatible with the standards generally accepted at the time of publication. Nevertheless, it is difficult to ensure that all the information given is entirely accurate for all circumstances. The publisher disclaims any liability, loss, or damage incurred as a consequence, directly or indirectly, of the use and application of any of the contents of this volume.

Copyright © 1988 by Appleton & Lange
Simon & Schuster Business and Professional Group

All rights reserved. This book, or any parts thereof, may not be used or reproduced in any manner without written permission. For information, address Appleton & Lange, 25 Van Zant Street, East Norwalk, Connecticut 06855.

95 96 97 / 10 9 8 7 6 5 4

Prentice Hall International (UK) Limited, *London*
Prentice Hall of Australia Pty. Limited, *Sydney*
Prentice Hall Canada, Inc., *Toronto*
Prentice Hall Hispanoamericana, S.A., *Mexico*
Prentice Hall of India Private Limited, *New Delhi*
Prentice Hall of Japan, Inc., *Tokyo*
Simon & Schuster Asia Pte. Ltd., *Singapore*
Editora Prentice Hall do Brasil Ltda., *Rio de Janeiro*
Prentice Hall, *Englewood Cliffs, New Jersey*

ISBN 0-8385-7204-9

Library of Congress Catalog Card Number: 92-083812

PRINTED IN THE UNITED STATES OF AMERICA

I dedicate this book to
my wife, Gloria, who has put up with me and all my papers all over the house,
and all the occupational therapy students who worry about passing the AOTA certification exam.

Contents

Preface *ix*

1 Gross Anatomy and Kinesiology *1*
   Explanatory Answers *19*

2 Physiology *31*
   Explanatory Answers *39*

3 Neuroanatomy *45*
   Explanatory Answers *48*

4 Psychiatry *51*
   Explanatory Answers *61*

5 Clinical Conditions *69*
   Explanatory Answers *80*

6 Evaluation *85*
   Explanatory Answers *109*

7 Planning *121*
   Explanatory Answers *152*

8 Implementation *165*
   Explanatory Answers *194*

9 Management/Administration *207*
   Explanatory Answers *231*

References *243*

Preface

This examination review book was written to give you a challenge in reviewing material that might appear on your certification examination for becoming a registered occupational therapist.

The first 400 questions are for reviewing anatomy, kinesiology, physiology, and psychiatry. These types of questions are no longer used in the certification examination but have been left in this edition for review purposes. If you have a strong background in these areas, the occupational therapy application questions should be easier to handle.

The 400 questions on occupational therapy are more like the questions asked in the examination indicated in the 1985 *AOTA Candidate Handbook*. These questions are generally longer than the examination questions but are written in this style to cover certain information or points of view. The corresponding answers are longer to give additional depth and breadth to particular points.

This fifth revision incorporates two changes: (1) it has reduced the non–occupational therapy questions to 400, and (2) over 100 new occupational therapy questions have been written in place of 100 that were omitted. Seven new books by well-known occupational therapists have been added to the reference list.

The reasonable answers given are from the references cited, which does not necessarily mean that all occupational therapists will agree with those answers. In looking at a particular answer and wondering why it is different from an answer you had in your occupational therapy school, you should be prompted to read the reference section on which the answer is based. This may broaden your view on this particular issue. Who is to say which "school of thought" was followed by the person who submitted the question for the national examination?

These questions were written with three thoughts in mind: (1) to give you some experience in answering a variety of multiple-choice questions; (2) to give you some incentive to ponder each question before deciding on an answer; and then, perhaps, (3) to take some time to read and study the reference from which the question was written.

Acknowledgments for this book go to the many excellent authors who have written the texts from which these questions were written. Additional acknowledgments go to Traci Jo Stacey and Julie Thorn who assisted in the typing of this fifth edition.

Notice

The author and the publisher of this book have made every effort to ensure that all therapeutic modalities that are recommended are in accordance with accepted standards at the time of publication.

The drugs specified within this book may not have specific approval by the Food and Drug Administration in regard to the indications and dosages that are recommended by the author. The manufacturer's package insert is the best source of current prescribing information.

The author has made every effort to verify thoroughly the answers to the questions that appear on the following pages. However, as in any text, some inaccuracies and ambiguities may occur; therefore, if in doubt, please consult your references.

The Publisher

1 Gross Anatomy and Kinesiology

QUESTIONS 1–5: On the left are listed common terms of position and direction. Choose the antonym for each term from the right column.

1. Anterior
2. Caudal
3. Dorsal
4. Proximal
5. Superficial

A. Cephalic
B. Distal
C. Deep
D. Posterior
E. Ventral

QUESTIONS 6–11: Match the plane with its definition.

A. A horizontal plane that passes through the body, dividing it into upper and lower halves
B. A vertical plane that passes through the body from side to side, dividing it into front and back halves
C. A vertical plane that passes through the body from front to back, dividing it into left and right halves

6. Sagittal
7. Transverse
8. Coronal
9. Horizontal
10. Frontal
11. Anteroposterior

QUESTIONS 12–15: Match the suture of the skull with its location.

12. Coronal
13. Sagittal
14. Lambdoidal
15. Squamosal

A. Between the parietal and occipital bones
B. Between the frontal and parietal bones
C. Between the two parietal bones
D. Between the parietal and temporal bones

QUESTIONS 16–23: Match the classification of joints with the number of axes about which it permits movement.

16. Ball-and-socket
17. Arthrodial
18. Hinge
19. Pivot
20. Ginglymus
21. Condyloid
22. Trochoid
23. Enarthrodial

A. Nonaxial
B. Uniaxial
C. Biaxial
D. Triaxial

QUESTIONS 24–27: Arrange the carpal bones listed below to read in order from the radial side to the ulnar side.

A. Lunate
B. Capitate
C. Scaphoid (navicular)
D. Pisiform
E. Trapezium (greater multiangular)
F. Trapezoid (lesser multiangular)
G. Triquetrum (triangular)
H. Hamate

	Proximal Row		Distal Row
24.	First	28.	First
25.	Second	29.	Second
26.	Third	30.	Third
27.	Fourth	31.	Fourth

QUESTIONS 32–36: Match the parts of the spinal cord with their features.

- A. Origin of the large nerves of the upper limbs
- B. Rootlets and nerves beyond termination of cord
- C. Termination of spinal cord
- D. Origin of nerves that supply lower limbs
- E. Tapering to a point toward distal end

32. Filum terminale
33. Cervical enlargement
34. Conus medullaris
35. Lumbar enlargement
36. Cauda equina

QUESTIONS 37–44: Select the **one** most appropriate answer.

---

37. The connective tissue that covers the entire muscle is the
    - A. perimysium
    - B. epimysium
    - C. endomysium
    - D. muscle fiber

38. The thickest and strongest tendon of the body is the tendon of the
    - A. iliopsoas
    - B. biceps brachii
    - C. gastrocnemius and soleus
    - D. teres major and latissimus dorsi

39. An increase in the anterior curvature of the vertebral column in the thoracic region results in
    A. kyphosis
    B. lordosis
    C. scoliosis
    D. spondylolysis

40. How many pairs of spinal nerves originate from the spinal cord?
    A. 12
    B. 24
    C. 30
    D. 31

41. The primary curves of the spine are
    A. cervical and lumbar
    B. sacrococcygeal and lumbar
    C. thoracic and sacrococcygeal
    D. thoracic and lumbar
    E. convex anteriorly

42. Rotation of the spine is most free in the
    A. cervical region
    B. lumbar region
    C. sacral region
    D. coccygeal region

43. The largest movable vertebrae are found in the
    A. cervical region
    B. thoracic region
    C. lumbar region
    D. sacral region

44. The vertebrae that can be distinguished by a foramen in each transverse process are the
    A. cervical
    B. thoracic
    C. lumbar
    D. sacral

QUESTIONS 45–49: List in order the parts of the brachial plexus from their origin to their termination.

45. First
46. Second
47. Third
48. Fourth
49. Fifth

A. Trunks
B. Branches
C. Roots
D. Cords
E. Nerves

QUESTIONS 50–60: Match the muscle with the nerve by which it is innervated.

A. Median
B. Lateral pectoral
C. Radial
D. Axillary
E. Musculocutaneous
F. Medial pectoral
G. Ulnar
H. Suprascapular

50. Pectoralis major
51. Pectoralis minor
52. Deltoideus
53. Supraspinatus
54. Teres minor
55. Corachobrachialis
56. Triceps brachii
57. Biceps brachii
58. Extensor pollicis brevis
59. Flexor carpi radialis
60. Flexor carpi ulnaris

QUESTIONS 61–66: The brachial plexus supplies the nerves to the upper limb. It is formed by the ventral primary divisions of the fifth to eighth cervical and first thoracic nerves. Match the nerve listed on the left with the first cervical or thoracic nerve that supplies it. For example, if the nerve is supplied from cervical nerves 5, 6, and 7, mark cervical nerve 5.

61.	Phrenic nerve	A.	Cervical nerve 5
62.	Axillary	B.	Cervical nerve 6
63.	Musculocutaneous	C.	Cervical nerve 7
64.	Median	D.	Cervical nerve 8
65.	Ulnar	E.	Thoracic nerve 1
66.	Radial		

QUESTIONS 67–79: Match the muscle with its insertion:

A. Coracoid process of scapula
B. Vertebral border of scapula
C. Bicipital groove of humerus
D. Deltoid tuberosity of humerus
E. Lateral third of clavicle, spine of scapula, acromion
F. Greater tuberosity of humerus

67. Trapezius
68. Latissimus dorsi
69. Rhomboideus major
70. Rhomboideus minor
71. Pectoralis major
72. Pectoralis minor
73. Serratus anterior
74. Deltoideus
75. Supraspinatus
76. Infraspinatus
77. Levator scapulae
78. Teres major
79. Teres minor

QUESTIONS 80–85: The muscles listed on the left act on the forearm. Match the muscle with the action for which it is responsible.

80.	Pronator teres	A.	Flexion
81.	Brachialis	B.	Extension
82.	Supinator	C.	Pronation
83.	Biceps brachii	D.	Supination
84.	Anconeus		
85.	Triceps brachii		

QUESTIONS 86–106: Select the **one** most appropriate answer.

86. The largest branch of the brachial plexus is the
    A. ulnar nerve
    B. median nerve
    C. axillary nerve
    D. radial nerve

87. Which cords of the brachial plexus are formed by the axillary nerve branches?
    A. Medial
    B. Lateral
    C. Posterior
    D. Anterior

88. The musculocutaneous nerve and part of the median nerve are the branches of the
    A. lateral cord of the brachial plexus
    B. medial cord of the brachial plexus
    C. posterior cord of the brachial plexus
    D. anterior cord of the brachial plexus

89. The difficulty encountered when trying to fully flex the fingers with the wrist fully flexed is called
    A. Codman's paradox
    B. tendon action of a two-joint muscle
    C. flexion paradox
    D. primary curve

90. The muscle most responsible for repositioning the thumb is the
    A. extensor pollicis brevis
    B. abductor pollicis longus
    C. abductor pollicis
    D. flexor pollicis brevis

91. The Purkinje fibers of the heart are the terminal fibers of the
    A. pacemaker
    B. sinoatrial node
    C. atrioventricular bundle (bundle of His)
    D. tricuspid valve

92. The lumbar plexus is formed by the ventral primary divisions of
    A. lumbar nerves 1, 2, 3, 4, and 5
    B. lumbar nerves 1, 2, 3, 4, and 5 and sacral nerve 1
    C. thoracic nerve 12, lumbar nerves 1, 2, 3, and 4
    D. thoracic nerve 12, lumbar nerves 1, 2, 3, 4, and 5

93. The common bile duct is formed by the union of the
    A. pancreatic and cystic ducts
    B. accessory pancreatic and pancreatic ducts
    C. hepatic and cystic ducts
    D. accessory pancreatic and hepatic ducts

94. For full abduction of the humerus, abduction must be accompanied by
    A. internal rotation of the humerus
    B. external rotation of the humerus
    C. flexion of the forearm
    D. supination of the hand

95. The iliocostalis, longissimus, and spinalis are branches of a muscle called the
    A. erector costalis
    B. semispinalis
    C. erector spinae
    D. splenius

96. Contraction of the entire trapezius will cause
    A. depression of the scapula
    B. flexion of the neck toward the same side
    C. retraction of the shoulder girdle
    D. rotation of the scapula

97. In case of injury to the musculocutaneous nerve, flexion at the elbow can be accomplished primarily by the
    A. extensor carpi radialis longus
    B. flexor carpi radialis
    D. brachioradialis
    C. brachialis

98. The movement that is performed at the wrist by the flexor carpi ulnaris is
    A. flexion
    B. extension
    C. adduction (ulnar deviation)
    D. abduction (ulnar deviation)

99. Abduction of the humerus is accomplished primarily by the
    A. anterior deltoid
    B. middle deltoid
    C. posterior deltoid
    D. pectoralis major

100. Outward (external) rotation of the humerus is caused by the
    A. anterior deltoid
    B. middle deltoid
    C. posterior deltoid
    D. infraspinatus

101. The short head of the biceps brachii has a common origin with the
    A. long head of the biceps brachii
    B. coracobrachialis
    C. brachialis
    D. brachioradialis

102. The enclosing membranous sac that aids the heart in maintaining its proper position in the thorax is the
    A. pericardium
    B. endocardium
    C. epicardium
    D. mesocardium

103. The medial and lateral plantar arteries are continuations of the
    A. arteriae dorsalis pedis
    B. anterior tibial artery
    C. posterior tibial artery
    D. plantar metatarsal arteries

104. The point of reference for defining abduction and adduction of the toes is the
    A. second toe
    B. third toe
    C. fourth toe
    D. first toe

105. The muscles responsible for abduction of the fingers are
    A. the dorsal interossei
    B. the palmar interossei
    C. the lumbricales
    D. all the intrinsics of the hand

106. The superficial component of the palmar aponeurosis is a continuation of the
    A. transverse carpal ligament
    B. tendon of the palmaris longus
    C. palmar carpal ligament
    D. dorsal carpal ligament

Gross Anatomy and Kinesiology / 11

QUESTIONS 107–116: Match the bone with its descriptive term or feature.

A. Ilium
B. Patella
C. Femoral head
D. Femoral shaft
E. Fibula
F. Ischium
G. Pubis
H. Talus
I. Calcaneus
J. Tibia

107. Second largest bone in the skeleton
108. Greater sciatic notch
109. Largest of the tarsal bones
110. Supports the tibia above it
111. Iliac spine
112. Fovea capitis femoris
113. Anterior part of innominate bone
114. Sesamoid bone
115. Linea aspera
116. Forms lateral part of ankle joint

QUESTIONS 117–132: Match the muscle with the nerve by which it is innervated.

A. Medial plantar
B. Tibial
C. Superior gluteal
D. Sciatic
E. Deep peroneal
F. Anterior branch of obturator
G. Inferior gluteal
H. Superficial peroneal
I. Femoral
J. Second and third lumbar

117. Tensor fasciae latae
118. Psoas major
119. Sartorius
120. Gracilis
121. Gluteus maximus
122. Rectus femoris
123. Semitendinosus
124. Adductor brevis
125. Gluteus medius
126. Gastrocnemius
127. Flexor digitorum longus
128. Tibialis anterior
129. Popliteus
130. Peroneus brevis
131. Extensor digitorum brevis
132. Flexor digitorum brevis

QUESTIONS 133–147: Select the **one** most appropriate answer.

133. The circle of Willis is an anastomosis of the
    A. internal carotid and external carotid arteries
    B. internal carotid and vertebral arteries
    C. external carotid and innominate arteries
    D. internal carotid and innominate arteries

134. Dupuytren's contracture will result in
    A. marked flexion of the elbow
    B. marked extension of the wrist
    C. marked flexion of the digits
    D. marked flexion of the wrist

135. The movement permitted at the elbow joint is
    A. flexion
    B. abduction
    C. adduction
    D. circumduction

136. The three scalenes originate on
    A. the first two ribs
    B. transverse processes of cervical vertebrae
    C. the second and third ribs
    D. spinous processes of cervical vertebrae

137. The muscles longus capitus, longus colli, rectus capitis anterior, and rectus capitis lateralis are collectively known as the
    A. strap muscles
    B. suboccipitals
    C. abdominal muscles
    D. prevertebral muscles

138. On which bone is a cribriform plate located?
    A. Sphenoid
    B. Palatine
    C. Nasal
    D. Ethmoid

139. The Y-shaped band at the front of the ankle joint is the
    A. superior extensor retinaculum (transverse crural ligament)
    B. lateral crural ligament
    C. inferior extensor retinaculum (cruciate crural ligament)
    D. flexor retinaculum (laciniate ligament)

140. A muscle that acts to prevent an undesired action of another muscle is
    A. a prime mover
    B. an antagonist
    C. a synergist
    D. a neutralizer

141. The thick fibrous band on the palmar surface of the carpal bones that forms a tunnel for the long flexor tendons and the median nerve is the
    A. transverse carpal ligament
    B. palmar carpal ligament
    C. dorsal carpal ligament
    D. lateral crural ligament

142. Movements of the shoulder girdle occur at the
    A. acromioclavicular and sternoclavicular articulation
    B. glenohumeral articulation
    C. scapula and clavicle
    D. scapula and humerus

143. The scapula is elevated by the
    A. upper fibers of the serratus anterior
    B. upper trapezius
    C. anterior deltoid
    D. middle deltoid

144 The same functions are performed by the teres minor and the
    A. teres major
    B. latissimus dorsi
    C. infraspinatus
    D. supraspinatus

145. The three vasti and the rectus femoris are collectively called the
    A. hamstrings
    B. intermedius
    C. quadriceps
    D. hipstrings

146. Pronation and supination of the forearm are allowed at the
    A. humero-ulnar joint
    B. humeroradial joint
    C. proximal radio-ulnar joint
    D. intercarpal joints

147. The fibers of the aponeuroses of the two obliqui abdominis and the transversus interlace to form the
    A. linea semilunaris
    B. tendinous inscriptions
    C. linea alba
    D. linea postscriptions

QUESTIONS 148–152: Match the type of contraction with the definition that most nearly describes it.

A. Gradual releasing of the contraction
B. Tension remains constant as the muscle shortens
C. Pulls the free end of the lever around the fixed point
D. No appreciable change in length
E. Muscle remains in partial or complete contraction without changing its length

148. Concentric
149. Static
150. Isometric
151. Eccentric
152. Isotonic

QUESTIONS 153–160: Match the muscle with its insertion.

A. Patella, tibial tubercle
B. Medial and plantar surface of medial cuneiform bone, base of first metatarsal bone
C. Greater trochanter of femur
D. Dorsal surface of base of fifth metatarsal bone
E. Lesser trochanter of femur

153. Psoas major
154. Gluteus medius
155. Peroneus tertius
156. Vastus medialis
157. Iliacus
158. Piriformis
159. Rectus femoris
160. Tibialis anterior

QUESTIONS 161–170: Match the bones of the skull and face with the descriptive terms or characteristics.

A. Sphenoid
B. Occipital
C. Temporal
D. Frontal
E. Lacrimal
F. Mandible
G. Ethmoid
H. Hyoid
I. Vomer
J. Maxilla

161. The smallest bone of the face
162. Light, spongy, cubical
163. Ethmoidal spine
164. Supraorbital notch
165. Foramen magnum
166. Horseshoe-shaped
167. Coronoid process
168. External acoustic meatus
169. Alveolar process
170. Forms posterior and inferior parts of nasal septum

QUESTIONS 171–177: Select the one most appropriate answer.

171. Receptors that transmit information concerning body position and movement are called
    A. exteroceptors
    B. thermoreceptors
    C. visceroceptors
    D. proprioceptors

172. Movement about an axis in which all parts of the object moving describe an arc is
    A. rotatory motion
    B. rectilinear motion
    C. circular motion
    D. curvilinear motion

173. Movement in which the object is translated as a whole from one location to another is
    A. angular motion
    B. translatory motion
    C. rotatory motion
    D. circular motion

174. The largest nerve in the body is the
    A. sciatic
    B. median
    C. femoral
    D. radial

175. What is known as the "funny bone" of the elbow is actually the
    A. median nerve
    B. ulnar nerve
    C. radial nerve
    D. musculocutaneous

176. The sacrum of the adult comprises _____ united bones.
    A. 3
    B. 4
    C. 5
    D. 6

177. The arteries and veins in skeletal muscles are found in the
    A. endomysium
    B. perimysium
    C. epimysium
    D. endocardium

QUESTIONS 178–187: Match the muscle with its origin.

A. Medial and anterior surface of the ulna
B. Distal fourth of the anterior surface of the ulna
C. Tendons of the flexor digitorum profundus
D. Lower two-thirds of the anterior surface of the humerus
E. Lateral epicondyle of the humerus
F. Middle third of the posterior surface of the ulna
G. Medial epicondyle of the humerus

178. Supinator
179. Flexor carpi radialis
180. Brachialis
181. Palmaris longus
182. Flexor digitorum profundus
183. Pronator quadratus
184. Extensor digitorum (communis)
185. Extensor pollicis longus
186. Extensor carpi ulnaris
187. Lumbricales

QUESTIONS 188–195: Next to each of the following bones of the skull and face, place the letter "S" if it is a single bone or "P" if it is a paired bone.

188. Mandible
189. Occipital
190. Parietal
191. Temporal
192. Sphenoid
193. Vomer
194. Ethmoid
195. Nasal

QUESTIONS 196–202: Match the muscle with the nerve by which it is innervated.

196.	Flexor digitorum profundus	A.	Median
197.	Flexor digitorum superficialis	B.	Ulnar
198.	Extensor digitorum	C.	Radial
199.	Lumbricales		
200.	Interossei palmaris		
201.	Opponens policis		
202.	Abductor digiti minimi		

Gross Anatomy and Kinesiology / 19

Explanatory Answers

1. (D) An antonym is an opposite. The opposite of each is as
2. (A) follows: anterior (ventral), front - posterior (dorsal),
3. (E) back; caudal (inferior), tail - cephalic (cranial, superior),
4. (B) head; dorsal (posterior), back - ventral (anterior), front;
5. (C) proximal (toward) - distal (away), the direction of a
limb toward or away from the center of a body; superficial - deep, the relative depth from the surface. (REF. 1, p. xvi)

6. (C) The sagittal, anteroposterior, or median plane is a verti-
7. (A) cal plane that passes through the body from front to
8. (B) back, dividing it into right and left halves. The horizon-
9. (A) tal or transverse plane is a horizontal plane that passes
10. (B) through the body, dividing it into upper and lower
11. (C) halves. The frontal, lateral, or coronal plane is a vertical plane that passes through the body from side to side, dividing it into anterior and posterior halves. (REF. 1, p. xvi)

12. (B) The coronal suture, nearly transverse in direction, is lo-
13. (C) cated between the frontal and parietal bones. The sagit-
14. (A) tal suture, placed in the midline, is located between the
15. (D) two parietal bones. The lambdoidal suture is located between the parietal and occipital bones. The squamosal arches posteriorly from the pterion and lies between the temporal squama and the inferior borders of the parietal bones. (REF. 1, pp. 297, 311)

16. (D) A nonaxial or irregular joint is irregularly shaped, allow-
17. (A) ing movement only of a singular gliding nature (non-
18. (B) axial). A uniaxial joint has a spoollike (concave) sur-
19. (B) face, which allows only a hinge-type movement about a
20. (B) single (or uni-) axis of motion. A biaxial joint has an
21. (C) oval, convex surface that fits into a reciprocally shaped
22. (B) concave surface. This allows forward and backward mo-
23. (D) tion but also some side-to-side action. When these movements are performed sequentially they constitute circumduction. In the triaxial joint a spherical head of one bone fits in a cup- or saucer-like cavity of the other bone, allowing for flexion, exten-

sion, abduction, adduction, circumduction, horizontal flexion, and extension and rotation. (REF. 4, pp. 578-579)

24. (C)
25. (A)
26. (G)
27. (D)
28. (E)
29. (F)
30. (B)
31. (H)

The proximal row of carpal bones is arranged in the following order: first, scaphoid; second, lunate; third, triquetrum: fourth, pisiform. The distal row of the carpal bones is arranged in the following order: first, trapezium; second, trapezoid; third, capitate; fourth, hamate. (REF. 1, pp. 371-372)

32. (C)
33. (A)
34. (E)
35. (D)
36. (B)

The filum terminale continues down the vertebral canal to the first segment of the coccyx. The cervical enlargement extends from the cervical to the second thoracic vertebra; it corresponds to the origin of the large nerves that supply the upper limbs. After the last thoracic vertebra, the lumbar enlargement tapers rapidly into the conus medullaris and toward its distal end. The lumbar enlargement begins at the level of the ninth thoracic vertebra and corresponds to the origin of nerves that supply the lower limbs. The collection of rootlets and nerves beyond the termination of the cord is called the cauda equina. (REF. 1, pp. 864-865)

37. (B) The concentration of connective tissue that envelops the entire muscle is known as the epimysium. (REF. 1, p. 506)

38. (C) The tendo calcaneus (tendon of Achilles) is the common tendon of the gastrocnemius and soleus and is the thickest and strongest in the body. (REF. 1, p. 608)

39. (A) The curvature at this level (thoracic) is a kyphosis. Other curvatures at different levels have different names. (REF. 2, p. 208)

40. (D) Thirty-one pairs of spinal nerves originate from the spinal cord: 8 cervical, 12 thoracic, 5 lumbar, 5 sacral, 1 coccygeal. (REF. 1, p. 1086)

41. (C) The thoracic and sacrococcygeal curves are called primary because they exist before birth; the cervical and lumbar

curves develop during infancy and early childhood. (REF. 4, p. 213)

42. (A) The cervical region contains the atlantoaxial joint, which accounts for 90% of the movement in the spine. The other joints are interlocked, and their articulate process thus is limited. (REF. 4, p. 224)

43. (C) The lumbar vertebrae are the largest segments of the movable part of the vertebral column. (REF. 1, p. 279)

44. (A) The cervical vertebrae are the smallest of the true vertebrae and can be distinguished by the presence of a foramen in each transverse process. (REF. 1, p. 271)

45. (C) The brachial plexus, as the name implies, supplies the
46. (A) nerves to the upper limb. The plan of the brachial plexus
47. (E) is as follows: roots, trunks, divisions, cords and nerves.
48. (D) (REF. 1, p. 1094)
49. (B)

50. (B,F) Anatomically and physiologically these muscles are inner-
51. (F) vated by the following nerve fibers: pectoralis major, lateral
52. (D) pectoral and medial pectoral; pectoralis minor, medial pec-
53. (H) toral; deltoideus, axillary; supraspinatus, suprascapular;
54. (D) teres minor, axillary; coracobrachialis, musculocutaneous;
55. (E) triceps brachii, radial; biceps brachii, musculocutaneous;
56. (C) extensor pollicis brevis, radial; flexor carpi radialis, median;
57. (E) flexor carpi ulnaris, ulnar. (All in REF. 3, pp. 17, 18, 21,
58. (C) 23, 25, 27, 30, 28, 48, 32, 34, respectively)
59. (A)
60. (G)

61. (A) The following nerves have their first roots in the cervical
62. (A) (C) or thoracic nerves indicated: phrenic nerve, C5; axil-
63. (A) lary, C5; musculocutaneous, C5; median, C6, ulnar, C8;
64. (B) radial, C5. (REF. 1, pp. 1094-1096)
65. (D)
66. (A)

67. (E) These muscles insert at these areas only, or their functional
68. (C) motion would be incorrect. (All in **REF. 3**, pp. 12, 13, 14,
69. (B) 15, 17, 18, 20, 21, 23, 24, 16, 26, 25, respectively)
70. (B)
71. (C)
72. (A)
73. (B)
74. (D)
75. (F)
76. (F)
77. (B)
78. (C)
79. (F)

80. (A,C) These muscles or combinations of muscles are the only
81. (A)   ones involved in the motion of the forearm. Each delivers
82. (D)   its force to accomplish its given task relative to the force of
83. (A,D) gravity or other neutralizing forces, preventing normal
84. (B)   function. (REF. 4, p. 116)
85. (B)

86. (D) The radial nerve is the largest branch of the brachial plexus. (REF. 1, p. 1101)

87. (C) The axillary nerve is the last branch of the posterior cord of the brachial plexus. (REF. 1, p. 1096)

88. (A) The musculocutaneous nerve is one of two branches formed when the lateral cord of the brachial plexus splits into two branches; the other branch is the median nerve. (REF. 1, p. 1097)

89. (B) A characteristic of tendon action of two joint muscles, such as the flexion of the fingers with the flexion of the wrist, is that all these muscles that flex in the same direction are not long enough to permit complete movement in both joints at the same time. (REF. 4, p. 49)

90. (B) By virtue of its location and its function at the wrist, it performs an action no other muscles can accomplish. (REF. 2, p. 152)

91. (C) The atrioventricular bundle (bundle of His) splits into two branches. The right bundle branch continues and breaks up into small bundles of what are called the terminal conducting fibers or Purkinje fibers. (REF. 1, p. 633)

92. (C) The lumbar plexus is formed by the ventral primary divisions of the first three lumbar nerves and the greater part of the fourth lumbar nerve with a communication from the twelfth thoracic nerve. (REF. 1, p. 1106)

93. (C) The common bile duct of the liver is formed by the junction of the hepatic and cystic ducts. (REF. 1, p. 1382)

94. (B) This action is possible only because the greater tubercle slides under the acromion, allowing complete abduction; other actions will not facilitate full abduction of the humerus. (REF. 2, pp. 103-105)

95. (C) The erector spinae muscle commences as a large mass in the lumbosacral region and divides into three branches: the iliocostalis, the longissimus, and the spinalis. (REF. 4, p. 233)

96. (C) Because of the wide origin of the trapezius its full contraction will only pull the shoulders back; contraction of parts of the trapezius will result in other actions. (REF. 2, p. 92)

97. (C) Other muscles cross the front of the elbow and are innervated by other nerves, thus allowing flexion to be accomplished. (REF. 2, p. 124)

98. (A) One of the three prime flexors of the wrist joint is the flexor carpi ulnaris, which will not flex the wrist or abduct it toward the ulnar side. (REF. 4, p. 131)

99. (B) The multipenniform arrangement of the bundles making up the middle portion of the deltoid gives it a potential for great strength and makes it a powerful abductor of the humerus. (REF. 4, p. 87)

100. (D) The infraspinatus muscle and the teres major acting as one combined muscle have two functions: to cause the humerus to

have outward rotation and to aid in holding the head of the humerus in the glenoid fossa. (REF. 4; p. 89)

101. (B) Each of the other muscles originates at a point other than the coracoid process. (REF. 2, p. 118)

102. (A) Although the heart moves freely and is not attached to the surrounding organs, it is maintained in its proper position, in the thorax, by an enclosing membranous sac called the pericardium. (REF. 1, p. 634)

103. (C) The posterior tibial artery, under cover of the origin of the abductor hallucis, divides into the medial and lateral plantar arteries. (REF. 1, p. 734)

104. (A) Abduction and adduction of the toes are away from and toward the longitudinal axis of the second digit, rather than the third as in the hand. (REF. 1, p. 500)

105. (A) The dorsal interossei abduct the fingers from an imaginary line drawn through the axis of the middle finger. (REF. 1, p. 590)

106. (B) The palmar aponeurosis is made up of two components: a thick superficial stratum of longitudinal bundles, which are the direct continuation of the tendon palmaris longus, and a thinner deep stratum continuous with the palmar carpal ligament. (REF. 1, p. 574)

107. (J) The tibia, situated at the medial side of the leg, is the
108. (F) second longest bone of the skeleton. The greater sciatic
109. (I) notch is a part of the bone called the ischium. The cal-
110. (H) caneus is the largest of the tarsal bones of the foot. The
111. (A) talus is the second largest of the tarsal bones and oc-
112. (C) cupies the proximal part of the torsus, supporting the
113. (G) tibia which is above it anatomically. The iliac spine is
114. (B) located in a part of the hip bone called the ilium. An
115. (D) ovoid depression on the head of the femur is called the
116. (E) fovea capitis femoris. The hip bone, or innominate bone, has as its anterior portion a section called the pubis. The patella, usually regarded as the sesamoid, is also called the knee

cap. The linea aspera, the posterior border of the shaft, is a prominent longitudinal ridge or crest on the femur bone. The distal portion of the fibula forms the lateral part of the ankle joint. (REF. 1, pp. 397, 382, 409, 408, 380, 391, 378, 397, 392, 404, respectively)

117. (C) Anatomically and physiologically, these muscles are inner-
118. (J) vated by these nerves as follows: tensor fasciae latae - deep
119. (I) peroneal; psoas major - second and third lumbar; sartorius -
120. (F) femoral; gracilis - anterior branch of obturator; gluteus
121. (G) maximus - inferior gluteal; rectus femoris - femoral; semi-
122. (I) tendinosus - sciatic; adductor brevis - anterior branch of ob-
123. (D) turator; gluteus medius - superior gluteal; gastrocnemius -
124. (F) tibial; flexor digitorum longus - tibial; tibialis anterior -
125. (C) deep peroneal; popliteus - tibial; peroneus brevis - superfi-
126. (B) cial peroneal; extensor digitorum brevis - deep peroneal;
127. (E) flexor digitorum brevis - medial plantar. (all in REF. 3, pp.
128. (E) 78, 62, 65, 70, 75, 66, 86, 73, 76, 92, 97, 88, 95, 100, 101,
129. (B) 103, respectively)
130. (H)
131. (E)
132. (A)

133. (B) The cerebral arteries originate from the internal carotid and vertebral arteries, which at the base of the brain form a remarkable anastomosis known as the arterial circle of Willis. (REF. 1, p. 691)

134. (C) Dupuytren's contracture operates at the distal end of the metacarpals and palmar ligaments and around the fibrous sheaths of the long flexor tendons. Thus, contractures in this area lead to flexion of the digits and nothing else. (REF. 2, p. 172)

135. (A) The articulations of the elbow joint allow only the movements of flexion, extension, and rotation, and, in some persons, hyperextension. (REF. 4, p. 113)

136. (A) The three scalenes originate at and run diagonally upward from the sides of the two upper ribs to the transverse process of the cervical vertebrae. (REF. 4, p. 237)

137. (D) The muscles known as the prevertebral muscles are the longus colli, the longus capitis, and the rectus capitis, anterior and lateral. The right and left muscles acting together flex the head and neck. Acting separately, they flex the head and neck laterally or rotate it to the opposite side. (REF. 4, p. 227)

138. (D) The cribriform plate is received into the ethmoid notch of the ethmoid bone. (REF. 1, p. 334)

139. (C) The inferior extensor retinaculum is a Y-shaped band placed anterior to the ankle joint. (REF. 1, p. 611)

140. (D) A neutralizer is a muscle that acts to prevent an undesired action of one of the movers. Thus, if a muscle both flexes and abducts but only flexion is desired in the movement, an adduction contracts to neutralize the abductory action of the mover. (REF. 4, p. 43)

141. (A) The transverse carpal ligament is a thick fibrous band on the palmar surface of the carpal bones, forming a tunnel through which the long flexor tendons and the median nerve pass. (REF. 1, p. 472)

142. (A) It is customary to define the movements of the shoulder girdle in terms of the movements of the scapula. In doing this there is some danger that the reader will visualize the movement as taking place solely in the joint between the scapula and the clavicle. It is important to emphasize that every movement of the scapula involves motion in both joints, the acromioclavicular and the sternoclavicular. (REF. 4, p. 90)

143. (B) The upper trapezius, the levator scapulae, and the rhomboideus major and minor help to elevate the scapula. (REF. 2, p. 98)

144. (C) The teres minor and the infraspinatus both arrive from the axillary borders of the scapula and are inserted into the greater tubercle of the humerus; thus, they perform the same function. (REF. 1, p. 571)

145. (C) The quadriceps or quadriceps femoris group consists of the three vasti and the rectus femoris. (REF. 4, p. 181)

146. (C) This joint is the only one allowing rotation of the head of the radius, which produces pronation and supination. (REF. 2, p. 158)

147. (C) The linea alba is the name given to a portion of the anterior abdominal aponeurosis sheath. It represents the insertion of the obliquus externus, obliquus internus, and transversus by the fusion of their aponeuroses with those of the opposite side. (REF. 1, p. 558)

148. (C) A concentric contraction occurs when the muscle actual-
149. (E) ly shortens and when one end is stabilized; the other
150. (D) pulls the bone and thus serves as a lever with the joint as
151. (A) its fulcrum. In a static contraction the muscle remains in
152. (B) partial or complete contraction without changing its length. Isometric contraction is a contraction without any appreciable change in length. An eccentric contraction is a gradual release of the contraction. The muscle actually returns from its shortened condition to its normal resting length. Isotonic contraction occurs when the tension remains constant as the muscle shortens. (REF. 4, pp. 38-39)

153. (E) The following muscles insert only at the area indicated;
154. (C) otherwise their functional motion would be different
155. (D) than normal; psoas major, lesser trochanter of femur;
156. (A) gluteus medius, greater trochanter of femur; peroneus
157. (E) tertius, dorsal surface of base of fifth metatarsal bone;
158. (C) vastus medialis, patella, tibial tubercle; iliacus, lesser
159. (A) trochanter of femur; piriformis, greater trochanter of
160. (B) femur; rectus femoris, patella, tibial tubercle; tibialis anterior, medial and plantar surface of medial cuneiform bone and base of first metatarsal bone. (All in REF. 3, pp. 62, 76, 91, 68, 64, 79, 66, 88, respectively.)

161. (E) The lacrimal bone is the smallest and most fragile bone
162. (G) of the face. The ethmoid bone in the skull is exceeding-
163. (A) ly light and spongy. The ethmoidal spine is a part of the
164. (D) sphenoid bone. The supraorbital notch or foramen is

165. (B) a part of the frontal bone. The foramen magnum is a
166. (H) large oval aperture at the base of the occipital bone.
167. (F) The hyoid bone was named because of its resemblance
168. (C) to the capital letter "U" (horseshoe shape). The
169. (J,F) coronoid process is thin and triangular and varies in
170. (I) shape and size relative to the overall size of the mandible bone. A part of the temporal bone is the external acoustic meatus. The alveolar process is a part of both the mandible and maxilla bones for the reception of teeth. The vomer forms the posterior and inferior parts of the nasal septum. (All in **REF. 1**, pp. 336, 334, 323, 333, 319, 317, 330, 315, respectively)

171. (D) Proprioceptors receive impulses from the tissues directly concerned with musculoskeletal movements and positions. (**REF. 4**, p. 62)

172. (A) Rotatory or angular motion occurs when any object acting as a rigid bar moves in an arc about a fixed point. (**REF. 4**, p. 282)

173. (B) Translatory motion means that an object is translated as a whole from one location to another. (**REF. 4**, p. 283)

174. (A) The sciatic nerve is the largest nerve in the body. It supplies the skin of the foot and most of the leg, the muscles of the posterior thigh, all the muscles of the leg and foot, and other parts of the leg. (**REF. 1**, p. 1112)

175. (B) The ulnar nerve, covered at one part only by skin and fascia, is called the "funny bone." (**REF. 1**, p. 1100)

176. (C) The sacral and coccygeal vertebrae in the adult unite to form two bones, five entering into formation of the sacrum and four into that of the coccyx. (**REF. 1**, p. 279)

177. (B) The arteries and veins in skeletal muscles are in a large vascular channel found only in the perimysium. (**REF. 1**, p. 506)

178. (E) These muscles have their origin in these general areas
179. (G) only, or their functional motion would be incorrect. (All
180. (D) in **REF. 3**, pp. 46, 32, 29, 33, 36, 38, 42, 49, 44, 59,
181. (G) respectively)

Gross Anatomy and Kinesiology / 29

182. (A)
183. (B)
184. (E)
185. (F)
186. (E)
187. (C)

188. (S) Of the bones of the skull and face, the mandible, occipi-
189. (S) tal, sphenoid, vomer, and ethmoid are single bones and
190. (P) the parietal, temporal, and nasal are paired bones. (All
191. (P) in REF. 1, pp. 315, 319, 331, 326, 322, 337, 334, 337
192. (S) respectively)
193. (S)
194. (S)
195. (P)

196. (A,B,F) Anatomically and physiologically, these muscles are
197. (A)   innervated by the following nerves: flexor digitorum
198. (C)   profundus, median and ulnar; flexor digitorum super-
199. (A,B)   ficialis, median; extensor digitorum, radial; lumbri-
200. (B)   cales, median and ulnar; interossei palmaris, ulnar;
201. (A)   opponens pollicis, median; abductor digiti minimi,
202. (B)   ulnar. (All in REF. 3, pp. 36, 35, 42, 59, 61, 52, 56,
respectively)

2 Physiology

QUESTIONS 203–209: Select the **one** most appropriate answer.

203. A respiratory mechanism sensitive to the lack of oxygen in the blood and lying adjacent to the aortic and carotid arteries in the chest is the
   A. apneustic center
   B. pneumotaxic center
   C. chemoreceptor system
   D. pressoreceptor system

204. Collapse of a portion or all of a lung is called
   A. asthma
   B. emphysema
   C. atelectasis
   D. dyspnea

205. In a normal blood pressure reading of 120/80, the 120 refers to
   A. diastolic pressure
   B. systolic pressure
   C. pulse pressure
   D. high blood pressure

206. One of the important substances that normally pass through the cell membrane by facilitated diffusion is
    A. carbon dioxide
    B. alcohol
    C. glucose
    D. water

207. The maintenance of constant conditions in the body fluids is known as
    A. mitosis
    B. hemostasis
    C. homeostatis
    D. nutrition

208. The average life span of the red blood cell is
    A. 1 week
    B. 20 days
    C. 1 year
    D. 120 days

209. The air that passes into and out of the lungs with each breath is called
    A. vital capacity
    B. lung volume
    C. tidal air
    D. residual volume

QUESTIONS 210–216: Match the part of the gastrointestinal tract with the digestive substance(s) it secretes.

210. Mouth
211. Esophagus
212. Stomach
213. Pancreas
214. Liver

A. Mucus
B. Hydrochloric acid
C. Amylase
D. Saliva
E. Sodium bicarbonate

215. Small intestine
216. Large intestine

F. Bile
G. Pepsin
H. Trypsin
I. Sucrase
J. Lipase

QUESTIONS 217–227: Select the **one** most appropriate answer.

217. Which diffuses through the pulmonary membrane most easily?
   A. Oxygen
   B. Nitrogen
   C. Carbon dioxide
   D. Alcohol

218. Muscle hypertrophy refers to
   A. extreme atrophy of muscle
   B. physical enlargement of muscle
   C. lack of exercise
   D. denervated muscle

219. Stimulation of the parasympathetic nervous system will cause
   A. decreased activity of the heart
   B. increased activity of the heart
   C. unchanged activity of the heart
   D. more rapid respiration

220. When arterial pressure is high, respiration is
   A. increased
   B. decreased
   C. unchanged
   D. fluctuating

221. The functional unit of the urinary system is the
   A. collecting tubules
   B. nephron
   C. renal pelvis
   D. urinary bladder

222. A high concentration of calcium in the extracellular fluid will
    A. increase the permeability of the cell membrane
    B. decrease the permeability of the cell membrane
    C. cause no change in the permeability of the cell membrane
    D. cause a great change in the permeability of the cell membrane

223. A solution that causes osmosis of fluid out of the cell into the solution is called
    A. isotonic
    B. hypertonic
    C. hypotonic
    D. hyperplasic

224. Which ions have the most difficulty in passing through the cell membrane by diffusion?
    A. Negatively charged ions
    B. Positively charged ions
    C. Neutral ions
    D. Ions with small atomic weight

225. The valve most frequently affected by rheumatic fever is the
    A. tricuspid (left atrioventricular)
    B. aortic
    C. mitral (bicuspid)
    D. pulmonary

226. "Edema" of a potential space is called
    A. effusion
    B. diffusion
    C. profusion
    D. infection

227. A trained muscle increases in size because of
    A. an increase in the number of muscle fibers
    B. the increased size of the individual muscle fibers
    C. increased strength
    D. increased efficiency

QUESTIONS 228–232: Match the five basic substances of protoplasm with their descriptive terms.

A. Provide inorganic chemicals for cellular reaction
B. Soluble in fat solvents
C. The fluid medium of all protoplasm
D. Plays major role in cellular nutrition
E. 10-20% of the cell mass

228. Water
229. Electrolytes
230. Proteins
231. Lipids
232. Carbohydrates

QUESTIONS 233–247: Select the **one** most appropriate answer.

233. Concerning the urinary system, the function of the glomerulus is to
   A. reabsorb from the filtrate those substances needed in the body
   B. remove the waste products of metabolism
   C. filter water and solutes from the blood
   D. increase filtration pressure

234. The simplest reflex arc is the
   A. axon reflex
   B. stretch reflex
   C. withdrawal reflex
   D. two-neuron reflex

235. The inhibitory transmitter secreted at some presynaptic terminals is believed to be the
   A. acetylcholine
   B. cholinesterase
   C. gamma-aminobutyric acid
   D. histamine

236. Once a single point anywhere on a nerve fiber becomes depolarized, a nerve impulse travels from that point
    A. toward a nerve cell
    B. away from the nerve cell
    C. in each direction
    D. toward the center

237. To vary the strength of a stimulus traveling down a particular nerve
    A. spatial summation is most often used
    B. temporal summation is most often used
    C. a combination of spatial and temporal summation is most often used
    D. one should increase depolarization

238. The presynaptic terminal secretes a substance that causes
    A. excitation of the postsynaptic neuron
    B. inhibition of the postsynaptic neuron
    C. either excitation or inhibition of the postsynaptic neuron
    D. inhibition of the presynaptic neuron

239. A nerve cell membrane suddenly becomes positive inside and negative outside. This is called
    A. membrane potential
    B. depolarization
    C. the resting state of the membrane
    D. polarization

240. The time during which the nerve fiber cannot transmit a second impulse until repolarization occurs, no matter how strong the stimulus, is called the
    A. action potential
    B. repolarization state
    C. action state
    D. refractory period

241. Interruptions of the myelin sheath at intervals along a nerve fiber are called
    A. the nodes of Ranvier
    B. Heberden's nodes
    C. the axoplasm
    D. unmyelinated axons

242. Most often the gradation of muscle contraction is attained by varying the number of motor units contracting at one time and by varying the number of times the muscle fiber contracts. This combination is called
    A. tetanized summation
    B. multiple motor unit summation
    C. wave summation
    D. asynchronous summation

243. The strength of muscle contraction can be increased by increasing the number of times the muscle fiber contracts. This is called
    A. tetanization
    B. temporal summation
    C. multiple motor unit summation
    D. wave summation

244. Which statement applies to the Purkinje system of the heart?
    A. Conducts the impulse from the atrial muscle latticework into the ventricular latticework
    B. Fibers transmit slightly more slowly than normal in rotating patterns
    C. Causes all portions of ventricles to contract nearly simultaneously
    D. Directs impulses around the heart

245. A drug that enhances the transmission of impulses at the myoneural junction is
    A. neostigmine
    B. cholinesterase
    C. curare
    D. acetylcholine

246. Alveolar ventilation is increased when
    A. carbon dioxide content of the blood is increased
    B. carbon dioxide content of the blood is decreased
    C. blood PH is high
    D. oxygen content of the blood is increased

247. In emphysema, which occurs?
    A. Collection of fluid in interstitial spaces of the lungs
    B. Total surface of the pulmonary membrane becomes greatly diminished
    C. Collapse of a portion or of an entire lung
    D. Increase in the alveolar walls

Explanatory Answers

203. (C) The chemoreceptors, neuronlike cells, are sensitive to the lack of oxygen in the blood and, when stimulated, send signals to the respiratory center to increase alveolar ventilation. (REF. 5, p. 214)

204. (A) Atelectasis is the collapse of a portion of the lung or of an entire lung. (REF. 5, p. 218)

205. (B) The blood pressure at its highest point during a pressure cycle is called systolic pressure; the lowest pressure is called diastolic. (REF. 5, p. 304)

206. (C) Glucose is one of the important substances that pass through the cell membranes by facilitated diffusion. (REF. 5, p. 511)

207. (C) For cells of the body to continue living, they have one major requirement, that of being maintained in extracellular fluid that must be controlled consistently day by day. This constant condition in these fluids is called homeostasis. (REF. 5, p. 5)

208. (D) Once the red blood cell has entered the circulation system, it circulates an average of 120 days, at which time it wears out and disintegrates. (REF. 5, p. 396)

209. (C) The air that passes into and out of the lungs with each respiration is called tidal air, and the volume of this area in each breath is called tidal volume. (REF. 5, p. 440)

210. (A,D) Saliva is secreted by the parotid, submaxillary,
211. (A) sublingual, and smaller glands in the mouth.
212. (A,B,G) Saliva is half mucus and is used to provide
213. (C,H,J,E) lubrication for swallowing. The esophagus
214. (F) secretes only mucus. The entire surface of the
215. (A,I,J) stomach is covered by a layer of very small mucus cells.

216. (A) The major digestive substances secreted by the stomach are hydrochloric acid and pepsin. The pancreas secretes about 1200 mL of fluid each day into the upper portion of the small intestine. Part of this volume contains amylase, trypsin, lipase for digesting food, and sodium bicarbonate for other purposes. The liver is the only organ that secretes bile. The small intestine secretes the enzyme sucrase; it also secretes lipase and mucus. The large intestine's only significant secretion is mucus. (REF. 5, pp. 497-505)

217. (C) Carbon dioxide has about a 20-to-1 solubility rate as compared with oxygen or nitrogen. Therefore, carbon dioxide can transverse the membrane more easily. (REF. 5, p. 446)

218. (B) The more a muscle is used, the greater it grows in size and strength. This physical enlargement is called hypertrophy. (REF. 5, p. 110)

219. (A) The vasomotor system helps to control the circulation through the vagus nerves, which carry the so-called parasympathetic fibers to the heart. When these fibers are stimulated, they decrease the heart's activity. (REF. 5, p. 272)

220. (B) Through the baroreceptor system, when the arterial pressure is high, the respiratory center is depressed and ventilation is reduced correspondingly. (REF. 5, p. 310)

221. (B) The main function of the kidney is formation of urine. The two kidneys contain approximately 2 million nephrons, which do the work of filtering out water and solutes from the blood. (REF. 5, p. 357)

222. (B) Permeability does not always remain exactly the same under different conditions. Excessive calcium in the extracellular fluid causes the permeability to decrease. (REF. 5, p. 594)

223. (B) When a cell contains a dilute intracellular fluid and is placed in a concentrated extracellular fluid called a hypertonic solution, water passes out of the cell by osmosis. (REF. 5, p. 68)

Physiology / 41

224. (B) Positively charged ions pass through the cell membrane with extreme difficulty because, it is believed, the positive charges on proteins or absorbed positive ions such as calcium ions line the pores and exert a sphere of positive electrostatic charge so that the two positive charges repel each other. (REF. 5, p. 73)

225. (C) Rheumatic fever most frequently damages the mitral valve. Rheumatic fever results from an immune reaction to toxin secreted by streptococcal bacteria. Antibodies formed against the bacteria attack the valves, causing growths on the edges of the valves which erode them. (REF. 5, p. 268)

226. (A) Edema of a potential space is medically called an effusion, although physiologically it is exactly the same process as edema. (REF. 5, p. 350)

227. (B) The greater size of a trained muscle is caused by hypertrophy of the individual muscle fiber and is not due to the appearance of new fibers. (REF. 6, p. 110)

228. (C) Water is present in protoplasm in a concentration be-
229. (A) tween 70% and 85%. Ions or electrolytes are chemicals
230. (E) dissolved in the water of the cell and are the inorganic
231. (B) chemicals for cellular reaction. Next to water, the most
232. (D) abundant substances in most cells are proteins, which normally represent 10% to 20% of the cell mass. Lipids are several different types of substances that are grouped together because of their common property of being soluble in fat solvents. In general, carbohydrates have very little structural function in cells but display a major role in nutrition. (REF. 5, pp. 23-24)

233. (C) The nephron, which forms urine from the blood, is composed of two major parts; one is the glomerulus, which filters water and solutes from the blood. (REF. 5, p. 365)

234. (A) The simplest neuronal reflex is the axon reflex. Other reflexes involve many more neurological functions. (REF. 5, p. 128)

235. (C) Some of the presynaptic terminals secrete an inhibitory transmitter instead of an excitatory transmitter. A large substance

found in inhibitory nerve fibers is gamma-aminobutyric acid (GABA), believed to have an inhibitory effect on the synapse. (REF. 5, p. 134)

236. (C) Depolarization is the opposite of polarization. In the normal polarized state, positive ions are located on the outside of the nerve and negative ones on the inside which keep a balanced depolarization in the opposite so impulses go in either direction as opposed to the normal balance. (REF. 5, p. 84)

237. (C) A nerve bundle has two means by which it transmits signals of different strength down a nerve: by simultaneously transmitting impulses over a varying number of nerve fibers, called spatial summation, and by transmitting impulses in small or large numbers over the same fibers, called temporal summation. (REF. 5, p. 92)

238. (C) Signals transmitted from the presynaptic terminals to the dendrites secrete an excitatory transmitter substance; other signals secrete an inhibitory transmitter substance. Therefore, some of these terminals excite the neuron and some inhibit it. (REF. 5, p. 134)

239. (B) The state attained when a nerve fiber membrane suddenly becomes positive inside and negative outside is called depolarization because in the normal polarized state the membrane is positive on the outside and negative on the inside. (REF. 5, p. 83)

240. (D) When an impulse is traveling along a nerve fiber, the nerve fiber cannot transmit a second impulse until the fiber membrane has been repolarized. This is called the refractory state, and the time during which the fiber remains refractory is called the refractory time. (REF. 5, p. 85)

241. (D) The myelin sheath covers all large nerve fibers and acts as an insulator around the nerve. Approximately every millimeter it is broken by a node called the node of Ranvier. (REF. 5, p. 82)

242. (D) Asynchronous summation is caused by neuronal circuits in the spinal cord that automatically distribute impulses among different nerve fibers to a muscle. (REF. 5, p. 109)

243. (D) Wave summation occurs when each muscle fiber contracts many times in rapid succession and close enough to each other so that a new contraction occurs before the previous one is complete. This makes each succeeding contraction add to the force of the previous one, increasing the overall strength of the contracture. (REF. 5, p. 109)

244. (A) Even though a cardiac impulse can travel perfectly well along cardiac muscle fibers, the heart has its own special conduction system called the Purkinje system that transmits impulses six times as fast as normal heart muscles, causing all portions of each cardiac muscle to contract in unison. (REF. 5, p. 261)

245. (A) At times a person has very poor transmission of impulses at the neuromuscular junction which may cause paralysis (called myasthenia gravis) from an autoimmune response, producing antibodies to the muscle membrane. Reaction of the antibodies depresses the responsiveness of the muscle fiber to acetylcholine. Treatment with neostigmine prevents the destruction of acetylcholine and overcomes the paralysis. (REF. 5, p. 94)

246. (A) The concentration of carbon dioxide in the blood is controlled by the rate of alveolar ventilation; however, if additional carbon dioxide is introduced into the blood, all portions of the respiratory center become excited. (REF. 5, p. 443)

247. (B) In emphysema, a disease caused most frequently by smoking, large portions of the alveolar walls are destroyed. Thus, the total surface area of the pulmonary membrane is greatly diminished. (REF. 5, p. 467)

3 Neuroanatomy

QUESTIONS 248–258: Select the **one** most appropriate answer.

248. Nystagmus is a term used to denote
  A. a nervous twitching of the mouth
  B. a burning sensation in the ears
  C. a rhythmic oscillation of the eyes
  C. a hypersensitive nose

249. In most instances a given sensory impulse terminates in the side of the brain opposite its origin as a result of decussation of the
  A. primary or first-order neuron
  B. secondary or second-order neuron
  C. tertiary or third-order neuron
  D. fourth-order neuron

250. Pathways from receptor endings to the cerebral cortex require a minimum of
  A. two neurons
  B. three neurons
  C. four neurons
  D. five neurons

251. The final common pathway is synonymous with the
    A. upper motor neuron
    B. lower motor neuron
    C. peripheral nerve
    D. motor unit

252. The pyramids, longitudinal prominences, are part of which portion of the brain stem?
    A. Thalamus
    B. Midbrain
    C. Pons
    D. Medulla oblongata

253. Surgical severance of the lateral spinothalamic tract for the relief of pain is called
    A. cordectomy
    B. thalamectomy
    D. cordotomy
    D. tractotomy

254. Which of the following sensibilities utilize the same pathway through the spinal cord and brain stem?
    A. Pain and somatic tactile
    B. Proprioceptive and thermal
    C. Thermal and tactile
    D. Pain and thermal

255. The dura mater is the _____ meningeal covering of the brain and spinal cord.
    A. innermost
    B. middle
    C. outermost
    D. thickest

256. Retrograde degeneration refers to the degenerative changes in the _____ stump(s) that occur after transection of a nerve fiber.
    A. proximal
    B. distal
    C. proximal and distal
    D. middle

257. Cerebellar, or intention, tremor may be observed in
    A. Wilson's disease
    B. parkinsonism
    C. poliomyelitis
    D. multiple sclerosis

258. Motor aphasia, or loss of vocal expression, is due to destruction of the motor speech area located in the
    A. inferior frontal gyrus
    B. anterior central gyrus
    C. posterior central gyrus
    D. cingulate gyrus

Explanatory Answers

248. (C) Nystagmus is a term applied to a more or less rhythmic oscillation of the eyes. One phase is called the slow component and is more prolonged; another phase is referred to as the quick component. (REF. 8, p. 103)

249. (B) The cerebral cortex requires a minimum of three neurons. The second neuron has its cell body in the posterior column of the spinal cord or in some nucleus of the brain stem and, with few exceptions, is a decussating neuron (i.e., its axon crosses to the side of the brain opposite its origin). (REF. 8, p. 47)

250. (B) Pathways from receptor endings to the central cortex require a minimum of three neurons. (REF. 8, pp. 45-46)

251. (B) This is the final common pathway because it is acted upon by six separate tracts and two reflex neurons and is the ultimate pathway through which neural impulses reach the muscle. (REF. 7, p. 188)

252. (D) The pyramids appear on the anterior aspect of the medulla as longitudinal prominences on either side of the anteromedian fissure. (REF. 8, p. 64)

253. (C) Cordotomy entails the surgical severance of the lateral spinothalamic tract at an appropriate level of the spinal cord for the relief of otherwise intractable pain. (REF. 8, p. 55)

254. (D) Pain and thermal sensibilities are served by the same pathway through the spinal cord and brain stem. (REF. 8, p. 52)

255. (C) The spinal cord inside the spinal canal does not fill the canal. The cord is covered from innermost to outermost by the pia mater, the arachnoid membrane, and the dura mater. (REF. 8, p. 29)

256. (A) Retrograde degeneration is the change in a cell body and parts of the neuron proximal to a trauma such as a cut. (REF. 8, p. 26)

257. (D) Cerebellar tremor is sometimes referred to as intention tremor. It occurs only during movement, intensifies at the termination of a movement, and is noted in multiple sclerosis. (REF. 7, p. 195)

258. (C) Motor aphasia is manifested by loss of the faculty of vocal expression and is due to destruction of the motor speech area, which is in the inferior frontal gyrus of the left hemisphere in right-handed subjects; it is also an indication of left cerebral dominance. (REF. 8, p. 133)

4 Psychiatry

Note: Wherever possible, the American Psychological Association's DSM-III terminology is used.

QUESTIONS 259–262: Match the humanitarian of the mentally ill with the country in which his/her reforms were carried out.

259. Chiaruggi
260. Pinel
261. Tuke
262. Dix

A. England
B. France
C. United States
D. Italy
E. Spain

QUESTIONS 263–265: Select the **one** most appropriate answer.

263. An early practitioner who used a method of treatment similar to, and the forerunner of, hypnosis was
    A. Jean Martin Charcot
    B. Liebault
    C. James Braid
    D. Anton Mesmer

52 / Occupational Therapy

264. The term "psychoanalysis" and many of its present-day techniques were originated by
   A. Charcot
   B. Janet
   C. Freud
   D. Breuer

265. The approach to psychiatry designated as "psychobiological" is credited to
   A. Freud
   B. Jung
   C. Meyer
   D. Adler

QUESTIONS 266–275: Match the three personality structures with their correct characteristics.

   A. Id
   B. Ego
   C. Superego

266. Contains compromising, solution-forming aspects of the personality
267. The "observing" portion of the personality
268. Operates on the "pleasure principle"
269. Concerned with such functions as perception, memory, and synthesizing experience
270. Attempts to adapt behavior to the environment
271. Acts as the repressing part of the personality
272. Collective name for primitive biological impulses
273. Operates on "reality principle"
274. Derived particularly from identification with parents and their substitutes
275. Demands immediate gratification of desires

QUESTIONS 276–281: Place the stages of personality development in the correct chronological order.

276.	First stage	A.	Phallic
277.	Second stage	B.	Adolescence
278.	Third stage	C.	Oral
279.	Fourth stage	D.	Latency
280.	Fifth stage	E.	Adult
281.	Sixth stage	F.	Anal

QUESTIONS 282–292: Match the experience or situation in personality growth and development with the correct stage during which it occurs.

A.	Phallic	D.	Latency
B.	Adolescence	E.	Adult
C.	Oral	F.	Anal

282. Concern arises about differences between boys and girls, especially in regard to sex organs
283. The individual is preoccupied with how he or she appears to others; there is a search for personal identity
284. Influence of authority figures outside the family provides opportunities for new identifications, as well as the interaction with a larger peer group in school/play associations and activities
285. Occupational choices or decisions are generally made
286. This period is essentially one of training in the customs and attitudes of society
287. Period of complete dependence
288. The individual independently pursues her or his own goals, with recognition of limitations and with willingness to seek advice from others when indicated
289. Aggressive drives may appear for the first time as shown in the pleasure of biting (appears in the last half of the stage)
290. Primary bond is between the child and the mothering figure
291. Power struggle between child and parent begins

292. Adult characteristics of dirtiness, obstinacy, and unreliability derive from this stage

---

QUESTIONS 293–312: Select the **one** most appropriate answer.

---

293. A false belief, not shared by others of similar background, that cannot be corrected by reason or logic because it forms in response to definite purposes and needs of the personality is called
    A. an illusion
    B. a delusion
    C. a hallucination
    D. disorientation

294. Disturbance in the flow of thought where both thought and speech suddenly cease is known as
    A. incoherence
    B. confusion
    C. blocking
    D. aphasia

295. Contradictory feelings and attitudes exist toward the same object: one of the two components remains repressed but may give rise to anxiety and feelings of guilt. This describes
    A. inadequate effect
    B. depersonalization
    C. ambivalence
    D. depression

296. Delusions of grandeur are an example of a disturbance of
    A. thought
    B. consciousness
    C. perception
    D. orientation

297. Amnesia is a disturbance of
    A. thought
    B. consciousness
    C. perception
    D. memory

298. Persistent and constant repetition of certain activities, which may be of position or body movement, is known as
    A. negativism
    B. dysactivity
    C. command automatism
    D. stereotypy

299. A perceptual misinterpretation is known as
    A. a delusion
    B. a hallucination
    C. an illusion
    D. a perseveration

300. Vivid recollection of minor details of a specific period of time or specific event is called
    A. organic amnesia
    B. psychogenic amnesia
    C. hypermnesia
    D. paramnesia

301. An illusion of memory, such as having previously lived through a current experience, is
    A. paramnesia
    B. hypermnesia
    C. jamais vu
    D. déjà vu

302. A person is akinetic and mute, but consciousness is relatively preserved, the eyes move, and respiration occurs. The person is thought to be
    A. intoxicated
    B. in a stupor
    C. in a dream state
    D. in a state of amnesia

303. Delirium is an example of a disturbance of
    A. sleep
    B. affect
    C. consciousness
    D. memory

304. During the psychiatric interview, questions about the ability to compare facts or ideas are used to determine the person's
    A. thought content
    F. judgment
    C. memory
    D. insight

305. Euphoria is an example of a disturbance of
    A. thought
    B. judgment
    C. affect
    D. perception

306. During the psychiatric examination, evidence of confabulation is noted as a disturbance of
    A. judgment
    B. behavior
    C. insight
    D. memory

307. Thoughts that persistently remain in consciousness against the conscious desire of the individual and that cannot be dispelled or influenced by logic or reason are
    A. obsessions
    B. compulsions
    C. delusions
    D. phobias

308. The firm belief by the patient that he or she has no brain, feels nothing, or is dead is included under the type of delusion called
    A. persecution
    B. grandeur
    C. nihilistic
    D. denial

309. Unrealistic fears that persistently thrust their way into consciousness and are accompanied by acute anxiety are
    A. obsessions
    B. compulsions
    C. delusions
    D. phobias

310. Delusions that give the individual feelings of perfection or special distinction are termed
    A. persecutory
    B. grandiose
    C. self-accusatory
    D. impoverishment

311. Korsakoff's psychosis is caused by
    A. vitamin B deficiency
    B. the toxic effects of alcohol
    C. hereditary factors
    D. an endocrine imbalance

312. Delirium tremens results from
    A. drinking over a period of many years
    B. sudden deprivation of alcohol in an excessive drinker
    C. an unusually severe or prolonged debauch
    D. malnutrition caused by drinking instead of eating

QUESTIONS 313–320: Three major types of clinical seizure are usually described. Identify the numbered statements (symptoms) according to the type of seizure.

A. Grand mal
B. Petit mal
C. Psychomotor

313. Loss of consciousness is sudden and complete
314. Episodic alteration of awareness associated with running
315. Electroencephalogram shows the focus at the anterior pole of the temporal lobe
316. Seizure includes tonic and clonic phases

317. Individual has a transient interruption of the stream of consciousness
318. Seizures tend to be accompanied by an increase in the speed and voltage of brain waves
319. The seizure may assume the form of a fugue
320. An aura is sometimes experienced

QUESTIONS 321–328: Select the **one** most appropriate answer.

321. A condition usually termed a variant of epilepsy and characterized by a sudden irresistible desire to sleep is called
    A. cataplexy
    B. narcolepsy
    C. catalepsy
    D. epileptic personality

322. Juvenile paresis is a brain syndrome associated with
    A. cerebrovascular disturbance
    B. infection
    C. endocrine and metabolic disturbance
    D. epilepsy

323. Cushing's syndrome is a brain syndrome associated with
    A. drug or poison intoxication
    B. intracranial neoplasm
    C. endocrine/metabolic disturbance
    D. infection

324. In early onset of a manic phase or in mild hypomanic cases, diagnosis of illness is most often based on
    A. cheerful, optimistic outlook
    B. poor judgment (e.g., excessive spending)
    C. abundant energy, mild excitement
    D. talkativeness

325. A mental disorder that includes paranoid delusions and in which the symptoms exist in two intimately associated persons (one with a primary illness and the other with an induced psychosis of a submissive and suggestible type) is called
    A. paranoia
    B. schizophrenia, paranoid type
    C. folie a deux
    D. involutional paranoid reaction

326. The cause of neuroses is
    A. anxiety
    B. fear
    C. conflict
    D. depression

327. Disorders of orientation may occur in any mental disorder. Disturbances of orientation are generally significant of
    A. acute cerebral insufficiency
    B. temporary inhibitions caused by preoccupation
    C. forgetting experiences as a result of psychological conflict
    D. conscious repression of one's time and place

328. Phenylketonuria is a condition associated with mental deficiency caused by
    A. trauma
    B. a metabolic disorder
    C. a chromosomal aberration
    D. psychosocial deprivation

QUESTIONS 329–334: Psychoanalytical therapy involves the following lettered items. Identify these items with the numbered items. The same answer may be used more than once or not at all.

A. Free association
B. Resistance
C. Transference
D. Countertransference
E. Interpretation
F. Dream analysis

329. The emotional reaction of the patient toward the analyst
330. The patient's inner tensions are expressed symbolically and disguised
331. The attitudes of the analyst toward the patient
332. An unconscious effort to evade
333. An uninhibited verbalization of everything and anything that comes to mind
334. Tentative explanations of patient's feelings and behavior

QUESTIONS 335–340: Four types of psychotherapeutic technique are listed. Match the technique and/or definition with the type of therapy.

A. Superficial expressive therapy
B. Suppressive therapy
C. Supportive therapy
D. Behavior therapy

335. Subtle suggestion; does not lead to real insight
336. Abreaction, emotional reliving of a stress situation
337. Emphasis is placed on controlling behavior through the "consequences" of that behavior
338. Used where immediate measures must be taken to relieve a patient (particularly when little is known) with unmanageable anxiety
339. Hypnosis
340. Narcosynthesis

Explanatory Answers

259. (D) The following people, humanitarians of the mentally ill,
260. (B) worked in the countries indicated: Chiaruggi, Italy;
261. (A) Philippe Pinel, France; Daniel Tuke, England; Dorothea
262. (C) Dix, United States. (REF. 11, p. 5)

263. (C) Mesmer's success with animal magnetic fluids and touching of his patients was short-lived, but this technique was picked up by an English surgeon named James Braid (1795-1860), who provided a descriptive formulation of mesmerism and introduced the term hypnotism. (REF. 11, p. 10)

264. (C) Sigmund Freud developed techniques of patient treatment, and from his careful clinical observations he constructed a system of psychology to which he gave the name "psychoanalysis." (REF. 11, p. 11)

265. (C) Adolf Meyer played a prominent role in the development of dynamic psychiatry in the United States. He insisted that multiple biological, psychological, and social forces contribute to the growth and determination of personality. He called this approach "psychobiological." (REF. 11, p. 13)

266. (B) Sigmund Freud postulated three hypothetical psychic
267. (C) segments in the structure of the personality called the
268. (A) id, ego, and superego. The ego (or "reality principle"-
269. (B) testing self) is that part of the personality that estab-
270. (B) lishes a relationship with the world in which we all
271. (C) live. The ego concerns itself with such important func-
272. (A) tions as perception, because it can mediate between the
273. (B) inner and outer world and attempt to adapt or com-
274. (C) promise behavior to maintain harmony between the
275. (A) urges of the id and the demands of the superego. The superego is conceptualized as the observer and evaluator of the ego function. It is derived particularly from identification with parents and their substitutes (figures of authority). These identifications are internalized and incorporated into the unconscious psychological structure of the child. Later in life the injunctions and prohibitions of other authorities are absorbed into the super-

ego, which then acts as a censor or supervisor of the ego and of inner unconscious tendencies and, therefore, as the repressing part of the personality. The id is a collective name for the primitive biological impulses. The psychologically determined drives for air, food, water, and other needs of the body and dependent longings, flight tendencies, and sexuality are thought to be the attempt to seek immediate gratification or pleasure (or the "pleasure principle" as it was called by Freud). (REF. 11, pp. 58-63)

276. (C) In psychoanalytical terms, the stages of personality
277. (F) development were thought to occur in the following
278. (A) order: oral, anal, phallic, latency, adolescence, and
279. (D) adult. (REF. 11, pp. 65-75)
280. (B)
281. (E)

282. (A) The phallic stage from about age 3 to about age 7
283. (B) shows a shift from the anal region to the phallic or
284. (D) genital region. In this phase concern is expressed about
285. (B) the difference between sexes and the presence or ab-
286. (D) sence of the phallic organs. This period seems to be
287. (C) resolved by mechanisms of identification in which the
288. (E) boy identifies with the father and incorporates the
289. (C) father's goals and standards into his own pattern of be-
290. (C) havior. In the adolescence stage from about age 12 to
291. (F) ages 20–22 the adolescent is preoccupied with how
292. (F) he/she appears to others and perceives himself/herself, called a "personal identity." One thing that happens during this stage is that the adolescent must commit himself/herself to a choice of intimacy with another and must make, as well, an occupational choice or decision. The latency stage of development, or later childhood, from about 7 to 12 years of age is so called because sexual curiosity is limited. In this period a child's socialization is regulated to others outside the family. In our Western culture these others include teachers and older and younger playmates. This period is also one of training in the customs and attitudes of society. The anal stage of growth and development from birth to 18 months, or longer in some children, is marked by the development of a primary bond between the child and the mother; it is a period of complete dependence of the child on the mother. After birth the child slowly moves to an "aggressive"

phase for the first time because needs are not met as comfortably as when "in the womb." This seems to be demonstrated or interpreted by the biting of a nipple in feeding. The adult stage is marked by independent pursuit of personal goals with a recognition of personal limitations and, further, a willingness to seek advice from others when indicated. During the anal stage motor development increases and the mother may focus on the child's effort to control his eliminative activities. If the efforts are made too soon and the child is punished for failure to comply, a power struggle may ensue. If the pressure to conform is not balanced, the child may evolve a pattern in later life of dirtiness, obstinacy, and unreliability from this stage of personality development. (REF. 11, p. 70-78)

293. (B) A delusion is usually defined as a false belief. But a false belief must be one that a person of similar education and experience would consider improbable or impossible and one that is not corrected in response to reason or logic. A delusion must also meet the definite purposes and needs of the personality experiencing one. (REF. 11, p. 129)

294. (C) Blocking is a disorder sometimes known as thought deprivation or thought obstruction and is often caused by some strong affect, such as anger or terror. (REF. 11, p. 129)

295. (C) In ambivalence, contradictory feelings and attitudes may exist toward the same object. Although only one feeling may be visible, the other is nevertheless present. The one that is repressed may give rise to anxiety and feelings of guilt. (REF. 11, p. 138)

296. (A) Delusions of grandeur or expansive delusions arise from feelings of inadequacy, insecurity, or inferiority. By using delusions or grandeur a person escapes from these feelings and, in his/her thoughts, achieves distinction and security. (REF. 11, p. 131)

297. (D) Amnesia may be produced by either organic or psychogenic factors. Organic disorder is caused by chemical alterations, trauma, or degenerative changes. In psychogenic amnesia, recall (for psychological reasons) is inhibited; that is, forgetting is not a passive loss of memory. (REF. 11, p. 144)

298. (D) In certain mental diseases, especially in compulsive reactions and schizophrenia, it may be found that when an activity has been initiated, there is a tendency to repeat it in the same manner for an indefinite period. This persistent and constant repetition of certain activities is known as stereotypy and may be of position, movement of the body, or speech. (REF. 11, p. 115)

299. (C) A perceptual misinterpretation is known as an illusion. Elements that are particularly likely to lead to misinterpretation of images are intense affective states, ardent wishes, urgent drives and impulses, and repressed elements. (REF. 11, p. 121)

300. (C) Hypermnesia is occasionally seen in mild manic states, paranoia, and catatonia. Impressions arising from emotionally colored events are registered with more than the usual intensity, with the result that the patient has a vivid recollection of details. (REF. 11, p. 144)

301. (D) Déjà vu is a feeling of familiarity with or prior observation of something that has not been previously lived through. It may arise when the present situation has an associative link with some past experience or occurrence for which the patient is amnesic. (REF. 11, p. 146)

302. (B) Stupor is defined as existing when a person is akinetic and mute, but consciousness is relatively preserved, the eyes move, and respiration occurs. (REF. 11, p. 142)

303. (C) Although it involves much more than a disturbance of consciousness, delirium is usually associated with infections, toxic states, metabolic disturbances, cardiac decompensation, or head trauma that impairs cerebral functioning and causes cerebral insufficiency. (REF. 11, p. 141)

304. (B) By judgment is meant the ability to compare facts or ideas to understand their relationships and to draw correct conclusions from them. Such questions and their answers assist in determining a person's judgment. (REF. 11, p. 200)

305. (C) A moderately pleasurable affect is known as euphoria. The euphoric patient is of an optimistic mental "set" and is confident and assured in attitude. Euphoria is often noted in hypomanic states and certain organic disorders. (REF. 11, p. 135)

306. (D) In a patient who shows impaired memory for recent events, the tendency to fill in these gaps of memory is called pseudoreminiscence or confabulation. (REF. 11, p. 145)

307. (A) Thoughts that persistently thrust themselves into consciousness against the conscious desires are known as obsessions. These thoughts may be strongly charged with emotions of guilt and are unwanted. As a defensive device, a guilty feeling of anxiety may be displaced by an innocuous idea, and the anxiety thereby decreases. (REF. 11, p. 133)

308. (C) Appearing at times with depressive delusions are nihilistic ideas when the patient believes that he/she has no brain and no feelings or that he/she is dead. Such ideas probably have their origin in vague feelings of emotional change and a subjective feeling of unreality or of changed personality. (REF. 11, p. 132)

309. (D) Like an obsession, a phobia thrusts itself persistently into consciousness. Morbid anxiety always accompanies a phobia, in contrast to the guilt or depression of the obsessed. The patient's anxiety becomes detached from a specific idea, object, or situation and is displaced to some situation in the form of a specific neurotic fear. (REF. 11, p. 133)

310. (B) Delusions of grandeur give the patient a feeling of escape from the troubles of reality that are too great a threat to emotional security. If the distress is guilt, he/she can secure perfection. If the patient has feelings of intolerable inferiority, he/she can have a feeling of distinction. (REF. 11, p. 131)

311. (B) Korsakoff's psychosis is one condition that results from vitamin B deficiency, a deficiency to which the chronic alcoholic is especially prone because of impaired gastrointestinal absorption, a diet largely limited to vitamin-free alcohol, and an increased vitamin requirement resulting from the high caloric effect of alcohol. (REF. 11, p. 325)

312. (B) The nature of the factors that operate in the production of delirium tremens is uncertain; however, it is generally thought to be a withdrawal syndrome precipitated by sudden deprivation of alcohol in the chronic alcoholic. (REF. 11, p. 628)

313. (A)
314. (C)
315. (C)
316. (A)
317. (B)
318. (A)
319. (C)
320. (A) A grand mal seizure is the most dramatic of the epileptic manifestations. Symptoms include the loss of consciousness, preceded by an aura in about half of the patients. After the loss of consciousness is the tonic phase of the seizure, which is followed by a clonic phase. Psychomotor seizures are characterized by many symptoms, one of which is epilepsia cursiva or "running fit." Sometimes the seizure may assume the form of a fugue. It is believed that the focus of electroencephalographic activity is the anterior part of the temporal lobe. There is an increased tendency to use the term temporal lobe epilepsy as a synonym for psychomotor epilepsy. The petit mal is the most frequent of the minor forms of seizure and is characterized by a transient interruption of the stream of consciousness lasting 5 to 30 sec. (REF. 11, pp. 278-282)

321. (B) Narcolepsy is described as a sudden irresistible desire to sleep. A patient, regardless of the situation in which she/he may be placed or of the activity in which she/he is engaged, may fall fast asleep. (REF. 11, p. 283)

322. (B) Juvenile paresis occurs in children or adolescents and is caused by congenital syphilis. It is transmitted from the mother to the offspring by the transplacental route after the fifth month of pregnancy. (REF. 11, p. 263)

323. (C) Interactions between emotional and metabolic processes may produce endocrine disturbances, and these, in turn, may affect cerebral functions and mental reactions. One of these is Cushing's syndrome; however, Cushing's syndrome is now regarded as the result of adrenocortical hyperfunction with either neoplastic or hyperplastic expression in the adrenal gland. (REF. 11, p. 312)

324. (C) A personality makeup involving episodes of a manic or hypomanic type often has, among other things, a simple depression following a manic phase and boundless energy. (REF. 11, p. 413)

325. (C) Clinical features of a "folie a deux" occur when one of two persons intimately associated with each other is suffering a paranoid delusion and this is communicated to and accepted by the other. (REF. 11, p. 453)

326. (C) Most major neurotic patterns are basically dependent on conflicting feelings and attitudes that arise in childhood. (REF. 11, p. 466)

327. (A) The process by which one apprehends his/her environment and locates himself/herself in relation to it with respect to time, space, and circumstances is known as orientation. If one does not recognize and locate himself/herself in these respects, he/she is said to be disoriented. Disturbances of orientation constitute the significant symptomatology of acute cerebral insufficiency. (REF. 11, p. 143)

328. (B) Phenylketonuria is the most frequently encountered and most thoroughly understood of the specific disorders of protein metabolism associated with mental deficiency. (REF. 11, p. 729)

329. (C) What is perhaps regarded as the most significant con-
330. (F) cept in psychoanalytical therapy, and perhaps the most
331. (D) important discovery of Freud, is the emotional reaction
332. (B) of the patient toward the analyst, known as trans-
333. (A) ference. The dream is regarded as a phenomenon direct-
334. (E) ly connected with psychic life. It represents a product of the person's thinking but serves as a convenient disguise for the person's unacceptable rejected emotions. In analyzing the dream, the analyst finds symbolic expressions of the patient's inner tensions and clues to repressed thoughts, feelings, and experiences. A phenomenon that accounts for many mistakes and failures of psychotherapy is that known as countertransference, transfer of the attitudes of the therapist to the patient. These attitudes can interfere with the therapeutic effectiveness of treatment but can be put to good use diagnostically and therapeutically. When the person is faced with emotional constellations with which he/she could not deal in the past that are repressed and forgotten and are about to be brought to light, opposition to their complete awareness appears. This opposition is known technically as resistance. Uncensored, uninhibited verbalization of everything and anything that comes to

mind is a technique used in psychoanalysis and called "free association." Another technique used in psychoanalysis is called "interpretation," wherein the therapist helps the person to understand the meaning of his/her mental phenomena and his/her behavior. (REF. 11, pp. 750-754)

335. (B) Suppressive therapy aims to strengthen repression and
336. (A) other usual defenses or to lessen the intensity of a disa-
337. (D) bling symptom using such means as suggestion and
338. (C) hypnosis. Superficial expressive therapy uses various
339. (A) techniques such as abreaction, which lessens anxiety by
340. (A) emotional reliving of the stress situation, and narcosynthesis, which uses an intravenous injection of Pentothal sodium to the point of relaxation (not sleep) so that censorship of unconscious material is lessened. Behavior therapies are founded on the premise that all social behavioral expressions, healthy or maladaptive, are learned or represent distortions or deficits in the learning process. This emphasis from learning theories on behavior as maintained and controlled by its consequences is now influencing the development of newer treatment methods. Supportive psychotherapy is anxiety suppressive. It seeks to diminish anxiety through reassurance, modification of the social environment, and the use of drugs. No attempt is made to produce insight. This permits respite and time for the restoration of personality organization. In many respects anxiety-suppressive techniques are similar to those used by many in crisis intervention. (REF. 11, pp. 763-769)

5 Clinical Conditions

QUESTIONS 341–351: Select the **one** most appropriate answer.

341. The chief indication for use of subarachnoid alcohol block for relief of paraplegic spasticity is
    A. severe pain immediately after injury and over the site of the injury
    B. the presence of motor and sensory function in the lower extremities, impeded by spasticity
    C. spasticity occurring within the first 3 months after trauma and impeding rehabilitation
    D. stationary intractable spasticity of the lower extremities, which have no useful motor or sensory function

342. The majority of patients with quadriplegia have lesions of the
    A. second and third vertebrae
    B. third and fourth vertebrae
    C. fifth and sixth vertebrae
    D. sixth and seventh vertebrae

343. The highest in incidence among the arthritides and those that exact the greatest toll in crippling are
    A. rheumatoid arthritis and rheumatoid spondylitis
    B. primary and secondary degenerative joint disease
    C. myositis and myalgia
    D. traumatic arthritis

344. The cardiac patient whose physical activity need not be restricted in any way is classified as
    A. A, class I
    B. B, class I
    C. B, class II
    D. C, class II

345. The condition that begins in the sacroiliac joints and spreads slowly upward causing fusion of the spine is
    A. ankylosing spondylitis
    B. Charcot's joint
    C. osteoarthritis
    D. villo-nodular synovitis

346. The first rehabilitation medicine service with its own personnel and beds of any civilian hospital in the United States was created in New York City's Bellevue Hospital in the
    A. 1920s
    B. 1930s
    C. 1940s
    D. 1950s

347. A person who has either suddenly or gradually lost his/her integrity, as in the case of a spinal cord injury or stroke, inevitably suffers from some degree of emotional instability. The physician or the health-related personnel must recognize that the most important factor in the first encounter with this person is
    A. taking an accurate history
    B. patience and understanding
    C. an ostentatious solicitude
    D. doing an accurate physical and mental examination

348. When there is a sudden stoppage of blood supply to a part of an organ with insufficient collateral circulation, necrosis of the tissue occurs. This is called
A. embolism
B. thrombosis
C. anoxia
D. infarction

349. When a person suffers a painful shoulder and also has certain conditions in the hand (slight swelling without pitting edema, increased skin temperature, pink glossy texture, and extension deformities in the metacarpophalangeal joints), which term is likely to be used to describe the condition?
A. Shoulder/hand syndrome
B. Peripheral nerve lesions
C. Rheumatoid arthritis
D. Rheumatoid spondylitis

350. An example of overproduction of bone, associated with greatly increased blood flow to the affected bones, is
A. Paget's disease
B. rickets
C. osteomalacia
D. osteoma

351. Loss of blood supply to a part of the body is termed
A. ischemia
B. anoxia
C. anemia
D. embolism

QUESTIONS 352–359: Match the different types of tumor, benign and malignant, with their descriptions.

352. Angioma
353. Sarcoma
354. Lipoma
355. Lymphosarcoma
356. Carcinoma
357. Myoma
358. Chondroma
359. Glioma

A. Malignant tumor of connective tissue
B. Benign tumor composed of muscle
C. Benign tumor arising from and composed of cartilage
D. Malignant tumor of neuroglia of the brain
E. Benign tumor of soft fatty tissue
F. Benign tumor composed of vessels as seen in a birthmark
G. Malignant tumor of the lymph nodes
H. Malignant tumor arising from the skin or from glandular organs

QUESTIONS 360–372: Select the **one** most appropriate answer.

360. The person with a very large face, protruding lower jaw, abnormally large hands and feet, and thick, coarse, furrowed skin has a condition caused by an overactive pituitary gland and called
   A. acromegaly
   B. Froelich's syndrome
   C. gigantism
   D. Simmond's disease

361. Hydrocephalus occurs when the intracranial pressure is raised as a result of blockage of the cerebrospinal fluid at the
    A. first ventricle
    B. second ventricle
    C. third ventricle
    D. fourth ventricle

362. Cretinism, a condition in which the person is dwarfed physically and mentally, is due to underactivity of which endocrine gland?
    A. Pituitary
    B. Thyroid
    C. Parathyroid
    D. Adrenals

363. One of the most important things a person can do to prevent decubitus ulcers is to
    A. learn proper positioning in a bed or chair
    B. use a foam rubber mattress
    C. use a sheepskin
    D. learn self-inspection for pressure signs

364. The Crede maneuver is a technique used with the paraplegic or quadriplegic to teach
    A. transferring
    B. bowel management
    C. shifting weight
    D. bladder management

365. A person needs an upper extremity prosthesis. Which component of the prosthesis is considered the most significant?
    A. Harness
    B. Stump sock
    C. Terminal device
    D. Hinges

366. The Muenster-type prosthesis extends posteriorly above the olecranon and intimately fits around the biceps tendon, thus suspending the prosthesis and eliminating the elbow hinges and triceps cuff. This prosthesis has achieved great popularity and is most often prescribed for the
    A. wrist disarticulation
    B. long below-elbow amputation
    C. short and very short below-elbow amputation
    D. long above-elbow amputation

367. From a purely functional point of view, the most desirable site of amputation of the upper extremity is the
    A. partial hand
    B. wrist
    C. short below-elbow
    D. long above-elbow

368. The first principle in treatment of disabilities resulting from lower motor neuron lesions is improvement of
    A. muscle strength
    B. eye-hand coordination
    C. hand dexterity
    D. range of motion

369. Terms such as exercise load, muscle load, and ten-repetition maximum are applied to
    A. resistive exercise
    B. passive exercise
    C. progressive resistive exercise
    D. active exercise

370. The most common cause of cerebral vascular accidents is
    A. hemorrhage
    B. embolism
    C. thrombosis
    D. compression of vessels

371. The incidence of emotional disturbance among the cerebral palsied is
   A. low
   B. high
   C. coincidental
   D. not determined

372. Which disease is congenital?
   A. Amyotrophic lateral sclerosis
   B. Tetralogy of Fallot
   C. Disseminated lupus erythematosus
   D. Diabetes mellitus

QUESTIONS 373–376: The numbered items are muscles that take part in movement. Match each muscle with its proper definition.

---

373. Prime movers or agonists
374. Antagonists
375. Synergists
376. Fixators

A. Muscles that oppose the prime movers
B. Muscles that stabilize the position of neighboring segments and maintain the limb of body in a position appropriate for carrying out the particular movement
C. Muscles that assist the prime movers and minimize unnecessary movement
D. Muscles that are essentially responsible for movement of the part

QUESTIONS 377–381: Select the one most appropriate answer.

377. If the physician asks the hemiplegic patient his name, the name of the hospital, and when he entered the hospital, he/she is doing an on-the-spot check of the patient's
   A. orientation
   B. memory and concentration
   C. perception
   D. emotional lability

378. Tetralogy of Fallot is a disease of the
   A. nervous system
   B. heart
   C. respiratory system
   D. liver

379. The hemiplegic patient who does not perform well in which of the following areas has the least chance to learn in a rehabilitation program?
   A. Tests of orientation
   B. Tests of memory and concentration
   C. Deficits in perception
   D. Emotional lability

380. Rickets, a disease of young children in which proper classification of bone cannot take place, is caused by a deficiency of
   A. vitamin A
   B. vitamin B
   C. vitamin C
   D. vitamin D

381. It is generally agreed that the elaboration of language occurs in the dominant hemisphere primarily because that is where the communication centers are located. The left hemisphere is the dominant hemisphere in roughly _____ of the population.
    A. 97%
    B. 90%
    C. 80%
    D. 75%

QUESTIONS 382–395: The numbered items are surgical terms. Match each term with its definition.

   A. Plastic surgery of the ear
   B. Incision of the colon
   C. Surgical removal of a lobe of any organ or gland
   D. Plastic surgery of the nose
   E. Excision of a gall bladder
   F. Removal of portions of the ribs in stages to collapse diseased areas of the lung
   G. Removal of a tumor or structure from its capsule
   H. Removal of part or all of the stomach
   I. Opening of a vein
   J. Excision of mastoid cells
   K. Renal incision for removal of calculus
   L. Removal of a lung
   M. Surgical creation of a gastric fistula through the abdominal wall
   N. Excision of a breast

382. Cholecystectomy
383. Colostomy
384. Gastrectomy
385. Lobectomy
386. Nephrolithotomy
387. Rhinoplasty
388. Gastrostomy
389. Thoracoplasty
390. Mastoidectomy
391. Enucleation
392. Pneumonectomy
393. Otoplasty
394. Mastectomy
395. Phlebotomy

Clinical Conditions / 79

QUESTIONS 396–399: The numbered items are clinical conditions or symptoms. Match the term with its definition.

A. Inflammation of a number of joints
B. Inflammation of the peritoneum
C. Pus in a body cavity, especially in the pleural cavity
D. Intoxication resulting from excessive thyroid secretion

396. Empyema
397. Peritonitis
398. Thyrotoxicosis
399. Polyarthritis

Explanatory Answers

341. (D) The subarachnoid alcohol or phenol block is the most useful method for relief of spinal cord spasticity. The chief indication for use is intractable spasticity of the lower extremities, with no useful motor or sensory function. (REF. 13, p. 342)

342. (D) The majority of patients with quadriplegia have lesions of the fifth or sixth vertebra. (REF. 13, p. 321)

343. (A) Rheumatoid arthritis and rheumatoid spondylitis are the highest in incidence among the arthritides and exact the greatest toll in crippling. (REF. 13, p. 562)

344. (A) Patients with cardiac disease who do not have limitations for walking, climbing stairs, lifting, or standing are classified as A, Class I. (REF. 13, p. 562)

345. (A) Ankylosing spondylitis is an unusual variant of rheumatoid arthritis. It begins in the sacroiliac joints and spreads slowly upward with bony fusions and calcification of the intervertebral discs. (REF. 12, p. 652)

346. (C) When the Rehabilitation Medicine Service was created in New York City's Bellevue Medical Center in 1946, it was the first such service in the United States and possibly the world. (REF. 13, p. 1)

347. (B) Personnel working with a patient who has suddenly or gradually lost his/her integrity and inevitably suffers some degree of emotional instability must recognize that patience and understanding are the most important factors in their first encounter. (REF. 13, p. 4)

348. (D) The loss of blood supply resulting from closure of an artery by thrombosis is called an infarction. It causes loss of oxygen supply to cells (which in turn die). (REF. 12, p. 114)

349. (A) Stroke patients have symptoms similar to those of people who have shoulder–hand syndrome. These should not be confused, because 5% of the people who have a cerebrovascular accident (CVA) also have a reflex dystrophy. This is characterized by a painful shoulder and a slight swelling without pitting edema in the hand with a pink glossy texture and a slight increase of temperature of the hand plus extension deformities of the metacarpophalangeal joints. (REF. 13, p. 609)

350. (A) Paget's disease of the bone is an example of overproduction of bone. The cause is unknown. It is associated with a greatly increased blood flow to the affected bones. (REF. 12, p. 649)

351. (A) Ischemia is a condition in which the blood supply to a local part of the body is diminished or stopped. (REF. 12, p. 79)

352. (F) The angioma is a benign tumor composed of vessels
353. (A) (usually blood vessels but sometimes lymph vessels). A
354. (E) birthmark is the most common visual sign of this disor-
355. (G) der. The sarcoma is a malignant tumor applied to con-
356. (H) nective tissue of bone, cartilage, fat, and muscle. A
357. (B) benign tumor of adipose (soft fatty) tissue is known as
358. (C) a lipoma. A malignant tumor of the lymph nodes is
359. (D) known as a lymphosarcoma. A carcinoma is the most common of all malignant tumors and may arise either from the skin or from glandular organs. A benign tumor composed of muscle is known as a myoma. The chondroma arises from cartilage attached to bone and is considered benign. The glioma is a malignant tumor of the glia or neuroglia of the brain. (REF. 12, pp. 301-302)

360. (A) An overactive pituitary that results in enlargement of the hands and feet, a markedly projecting lower jaw, and thick, coarse, furrowed skin is diagnosed as acromegaly. (REF. 12, p. 546)

361. (D) When the cerebrospinal fluid cannot escape the fourth ventricle, it accumulates and distends the ventricles, pressing against the skull. This condition is called hydrocephalus or water on the brain. (REF. 12, p. 608)

362. (B) A cretin is an individual in whom the thyroid has failed to develop, resulting in an underdeveloped body and brain. (REF. 12, p. 559)

363. (D) The person with a decubitus ulcer should examine his/her skin daily to detect reddened areas. Taking the necessary precautions after such detection is one of the most important things the person can do to prevent an ulcer. (REF. 13, p. 250)

364. (D) Urologic rehabilitation of the person with paraplegia is directed toward complete or nearly complete evacuation of the bladder. One way to aid this is by the Crede maneuver. (REF. 13, p. 353)

365. (C) The most significant component of the upper extremity prosthesis is the terminal device, which provides either function or cosmesis. (REF. 15, p. 498)

366. (C) For the short and very short below-elbow amputee, the Muenster-type prosthesis has achieved great popularity; however, it limits elbow flexion and extension. (REF. 13, p. 240)

367. (B) Wrist disarticulation is more desirable from a functional point of view, since with the prosthesis the person would retain nearly full pronation-supination as well as other ranges of motions. (REF. 13, p. 239)

368. (A) The first principle in treatment of disabilities resulting from lower motor neuron lesions is improvement of muscle strength using appropriate activities to encourage active motion. (REF. 13, p. 124)

369. (C) Progressive resistive exercise, which is employed primarily for strengthening a muscle group, utilizes muscle load, ten-repetition maximum/minimum, and other concepts. (REF. 13, p. 101)

370. (C) A thrombosis is the most common cause of a cerebral vascular accident, or stroke. (REF. 12, p. 612)

371. (B) Despite widespread opinion, there is no solid evidence that different types of cerebral palsy are associated with different personality characteristics; however, emotional disturbance in this group is high. (REF. 13, p. 29)

372. (B) Tetralogy of Fallot is the most important congenital lesion of the heart and the most common one causing cyanosis. (REF. 12, p. 354)

373. (D) Prime movers or agonists are those muscles that are es-
374. (A) sentially responsible for movement of the part. An-
375. (C) tagonists are those muscles that oppose the prime
376. (B) movers. Synergists are those muscles that assist the prime movers and minimize unnecessary movement. Fixator muscles are those that stabilize the position of neighboring segments and maintain the limb or body in a position appropriate for carrying out the particular movement needed. (REF. 13, p. 96)

377. (A) Several fairly rapid techniques for assessing various areas of mental dysfunction are available. One for orientation includes asking the subject name, name or location of the hospital, current date, and date of entrance into the hospital. (REF. 13, p. 26)

378. (B) Tetralogy of Fallot is a congenital lesion of the heart. (REF. 12, p. 354)

379. (C) Patients who are found to have the best indices of how well they can learn in a rehabilitation program are those that do best in perceptual tests. (REF. 13, p. 27)

380. (D) Rickets is a form of osteodystrophy that is a manifestation of a vitamin D deficiency. (REF. 12, p. 86)

381. (A) In roughly 97% of the population, the left hemisphere of the brain is the dominant hemisphere. Hence the close association is made between language pathology and right-sided motor and sensory impairment. (REF. 13, p. 261)

382. (E) Cholecystectomy is removal of the gall bladder.
383. (B) Colostomy is an incision of the colon. Gastrectomy is
384. (H) surgical removal of part or all of the stomach. Lobec-
385. (C) tomy is surgical removal of a lobe or any organ or
386. (K) gland. Nephrolithotomy is a renal incision for removal
387. (D) of calculus. Rhinoplasty is plastic surgery of the nose.
388. (M) Gastrostomy is surgical creation of a gastric fistula

389. (F) through the abdominal wall. A thoracoplasty upon the
390. (J) thorax is removal of portions of the ribs in stages to
391. (G) collapse diseased areas of the lung. A mastoidectomy is
392. (L) the excision of mastoid cells. Enucleation is removal of
393. (A) the tumor or structure from its capsule. Pneumonec-
394. (N) tomy is surgical removal of a lung. Otoplasty is plastic
395. (I) surgery of the ear to correct defects. Mastectomy is excision of one or both breasts. Phlebotomy is the opening of a vein. (All in REF. 14, pp. C-59, C-92, G-10, L-48, N-13, R-45, G-14, T-33, M-15, E-40, P-99, O-37, M-14, P-70, respectively)

396. (C) Empyema is pus in a body cavity, especially in the
397. (B) pleural cavity. Peritonitis is inflammation of the
398. (D) peritoneum. Thyrotoxicosis is a condition of intoxica-
399. (A) tion resulting from excessive thyroid secretion. Polyarthritis is inflammation of a number of joints. (All in REF. 14, pp. E-24, P-56, T-41, P-110, respectively)

6 Evaluation

QUESTIONS 400–442: Select the **one** most appropriate answer.

400. In the evaluation of a person for an occupational therapy program, initial assessments of self-maintenance include
    A. person's income pre- and post-hospitalization
    B. ability to handle tools and fix things around the house
    C. activities needed to maintain life support needs
    D. ability to handle the activities given in occupational therapy

401. In the evaluation of a person for an occupational therapy program, initial assessments of productivity include
    A. how many articles a person can make during a week's time
    B. ability to follow directions, use judgment, be punctual, and exercise certain skills
    C. mental capacity in producing written and verbal answers to test questions
    D. ability to produce verbal and social skills in an interview, group setting, and staffing

86 / Occupational Therapy

402. In the evaluation for occupational therapy of a person's leisure time utilization, the therapist examines
    A. the types of activities a person does for enjoyment
    B. how much time is spent on leisure versus work
    C. the amount of time spent on leisure versus work or rest/sleep
    D. how much time is spent with other people versus individual activity

403. The motor component of performance is evaluated prior to occupational therapy to determine if
    A. the person can get to occupational therapy without any help
    B. muscle strength and range of motion (ROM) are within normal range for the illness
    C. the person has the basic skills needed to complete occupational requirements
    D. the neuromuscular/skeletal system is able to withstand movement from the bed to occupational therapy for treatment

404. The sensory component of performance is evaluated by an occupational therapist to determine
    A. if the person has any sense
    B. if senses are able to function separately and cooperatively and with the motor components
    C. if the person can tolerate all the input in an occupational therapy setting
    D. at what level the senses are able to function separately along with an evaluation of motor component

405. The cognitive component of performance is evaluated to establish patients'
    A. knowledge about where they are, what day it is, and what year it is
    B. ability to recall name, age, and past and recent events
    C. ability to learn a task, solve a problem, and remember skills for short and long periods
    D. knowledge about themselves in order to share and profit from treatment in occupational therapy

406. The intrapersonal component of performance is assessed by the therapist to determine
   A. the ability of the person to distinguish reality from unreality and to cope with that reality
   B. the group to which the person should be assigned
   C. if the person is able to relate to other people
   D. if and how long the person should be assigned to occupational therapy

407. The interpersonal component of performance is measured by the therapist to determine
   A. if the person is able to relate to other people
   B. the ability of the person to distinguish reality from unreality and to cope with that reality
   C. the group to which the person should be assigned
   D. if and how long the person should be assigned to occupational therapy

408. Evaluation is basically used to determine a person's level of occupational performance skill and functional ability both present and past. The therapist in an initial or screening evaluation should
   A. determine the past and current levels of function due to conditions presenting the patient to occupational therapy
   B. determine what functions are slow and regressed to speed up treatment procedures
   C. pay attention to normal and above-normal performance as well as to dysfunctions (past and present)
   D. pay special attention to the ability a person demonstrates in activities offered in occupational therapy

409. The primary purpose of an evaluation is to
   A. develop rapport with the person
   B. gather, analyze, and interpret data
   C. get to know the person and plan a treatment program schedule
   D. plan tests and procedures to use

410. Learning about a child prior to an evaluation
    A. has advantages and disadvantages
    B. is completely immaterial
    C. is relative to an institution's procedure
    D. is relative to your own procedure

411. Through a study of the child's reported developmental history, the therapist, prior to the child coming to occupational therapy,
    A. knows what is wrong with the child
    B. is guided in choosing the evaluation process to be used
    C. plans a treatment program
    D. consults with the referring physician before seeing the child

412. From a developmental history the therapist learns that a child performs developmental tasks within a 2- to 3-year-old range although the child is 6 years old. The therapist will choose an evaluation that incorporates tasks
    A. from 6 months to 6 years
    B. from about 1-1/2 to 4 years
    C. from 3 months to 8 years
    D. from 2 to 3 years

413. Precautions and restrictions noted on a patient's record provide the therapist with information so that the therapist can
    A. look for these behaviors to chart
    B. have the rest of the staff alerted in case of problems
    C. expect the unexpected and function more confidently
    D. go to the ward and see the patient first to know for sure what is happening

414. Skillful interviewing can smooth the way for ongoing parent-therapist communication. No matter what the content of the interview, the primary objective is to
   A. let the family know that the therapist is a professional and knows how to handle the problem
   B. let the family know what will take place in the treatment process
   C. show the family that, no matter what the cost, the treatment will be successful
   D. show the family that the therapist is genuinely interested in the problem

415. In keeping a therapist's work current, evaluation (or rather reevaluation) should be assessed and each target area reviewed because
   A. the profession lacks research and each evaluation would serve to support the technique or procedure used
   B. the therapist needs this protection to keep from becoming involved with any future litigation
   C. the therapist needs to determine the effectiveness of the activity process and to revise the objectives as they are mastered by the patient
   D. the patient needs to be assured that the therapist is performing treatment adequately

416. In the interview, one of several evaluation processes, the therapist must have a solid knowledge base to
   A. let the person and/or family know that the therapist is a professional
   B. let the interview report show what questions were asked
   C. plan a treatment plan simultaneously with the gathering of data from the person in order to save time
   D. select questions or areas to be covered

417. Manual muscle testing is a procedure in which the strength of a muscle is determined through manual evaluation. In this test, the therapist has the patient move the part through
    A. the full range of motion with gravity eliminated
    B. the full range of motion against gravity
    C. the full range of motion against gravity and resistance
    D. the full range of motion against gravity and then against gravity and resistance

418. In manual muscle testing using a grading scale of 5 to 0 and/or N-Normal to 0-Zero, a rating of F-Fair or 3 is recorded. This rating is a complete ROM
    A. against gravity with full resistance
    B. against gravity with some resistance
    C. against gravity
    D. with gravity eliminated

419. In the evaluation of ROM the goniometer is the most frequently used tool. The procedure that maintains the highest reliability and accuracy each time the person is measured is to use the same therapist
    A. and the same method at the same time of day
    B. and the same method whenever the person is relaxed
    C. and the same method when the person is fully relaxed and only when the person is flat on her or his back
    D. and any method at any time of day

420. The evaluation of sensation, ROM, muscle tone, reflex development and integration, sensory-motor development, strength, endurance, and coordination is used when the person has
    A. a psychotic dysfunction
    B. a central nervous system dysfunction
    C. an orthopedic dysfunction
    D. an immune defense system dysfunction

421. In the evaluation of muscle tone, the resistance a muscle offers to passive stretch, which is used to evaluate muscle tone on an extremity, is
    A. active movement
    B. passive movement
    C. active resistive movement
    D. active assistive movement

422. If muscle tone is increased, which will occur in an extremity as a result of passive movement?
    A. No difference
    B. Decreased resistance
    C. Increased resistance
    D. Free movement

423. In the evaluation of reflex testing one should remember that reflex responses to stimuli develop in fetal life and continue to dominate motor behavior through and not too far beyond
    A. early infancy
    B. childhood
    C. early adolescence
    D. late adolescence

424. Reflexes are tested by applying the appropriate stimulus and observing the response. If the reflex response occurs, the reflex is positive; if not, it is negative. No conclusion can be made from a positive or negative response unless the therapist knows
    A. the diagnosis
    B. the degree of positive or negative reaction
    C. the limits of the disease process
    D. the age of the individual

425. The grasp reflex in a normal baby from birth to 3 or 4 months shows finger flexion and a strong grip that persists and resists removal of the stimulus object. This action occurs when the therapist, in evaluating the child, applies pressure to the
   A. tips of the fingers
   B. thumb and fingers
   C. palm of the hand on the ulnar side
   D. palm of the hand on the radial side

426. In the evaluation of a spinal level reflex in a normal child up to 2 months of age, the therapist places the child in a supine position with the head in midline and the legs extended. A quick tactile stimulus is applied to the sole of the foot. Which response will take place in that leg?
   A. A quick knee jerk
   B. A full extension of the toes
   C. An uncontrolled flexion of the leg
   D. An uncontrolled extension of the leg

427. In the evaluation discussed in Question 426, the child is in the same position except one leg is extended and the other leg is fully flexed. The therapist applies pressure to the ball of the foot of the flexed leg. Which response will take place in the flexed leg?
   A. A quick knee jerk
   B. A full extension of the toes
   C. An uncontrolled flexion of the leg
   D. An uncontrolled extension of the leg

428. With the child in Questions 426 and 427 in a supine position with the head in midposition, one leg extended, and the other leg fully flexed, which response will occur when the extended leg is passively flexed?
   A. Extension of the opposite leg with hip adduction on internal rotation
   B. Extension of the stimulated leg with hip adduction and internal rotation
   C. Flexion of the opposite leg with hip adduction and internal rotation
   D. Flexion of the stimulated leg with hip adduction and internal rotation

429. A child is supine with the head in midposition and both legs extended. The adduction surface of one thigh is stimulated and hip adduction and internal rotation of the opposite leg occur. To which outcome will evaluation of this child lead?
   A. Hip extension tightness or spasticity exists
   B. Hip flexor tightness or spasticity exists
   C. Knee extension tightness or spasticity exists
   D. Knee extension tightness or spasticity exists

430. For most normal babies with strong reflexes, from birth to 4 months, who are in the supine position with arms and legs extended, if the therapist either passively or actively turns the head 90 degrees to one side, which observation will be made?
   A. Flexion of the limbs on the face side and flexion of the limbs on the skull side
   B. Flexion of the limbs on the face side and extension of the limbs on the skull side
   C. Extension of the limbs on the face side and extension of the limbs on the skull side
   D. Extension of the limbs on the face side and flexion of the limbs on the skull side

94 / Occupational Therapy

431. A normal child from birth to 4 months is placed in the prone position with the head in midposition, and flexion of the extremities or increased flexor tone is observed. Which stimulus produced this behavior?
    A. Pressure on the balls of both feet
    B. Pressure on the ball of one foot
    C. Scraping a sharp object from the heel to the ball of the foot
    D. Placement of the child in this position

432. The "Bobath reaction" in a normal child from birth to 6 months placed in the supine position with arms and legs extended results in which response when the head is passively turned to one side and held in that position?
    A. The child tries to go in the opposite direction from the head
    B. The child turns in the direction of the head
    C. The child's arms and legs immediately flex
    D. The child's arms and legs go into hyperextension

433. When the child described in Question 432 is past 6 months, up to age 4 or 5 years, and is placed in the same position and the therapist uses the same action, what is the result?
    A. The whole body will smoothly follow the head direction
    B. The whole body will smoothly follow in the opposite direction
    C. The body will follow a segmental rotation around the body axis in the same direction
    D. The body will follow a segmental rotation around the body axis in the opposite direction

434. Standardized tests provide normative data on specific behavior of a specific population. To obtain valid results, the therapist
    A. can follow any procedure as long as all questions are asked
    B. must follow the procedures stipulated
    C. must ask all questions but in his/her own way
    D. can ask any question as long as the content is the same

435. In scoring and/or analyzing a standardized test, to obtain valid results a therapist must
    A. follow any procedure as long as all questions are given the same consideration in scoring them
    B. follow the procedures stipulated
    C. score all questions using the same logic
    D. score all questions taking into consideration the patient's ability and dysfunction

436. Tests administered in occupational therapy in the evaluation of a person prior to treatment
    A. can be administered by an occupational therapist, registered (OTR)
    B. can be administered by an OTR or a certified occupational therapy assistant (COTA)
    C. may require special training
    D. may require special training and certification

437. When a therapist needs to evaluate a child's sensory integrative and motor functions, data should be recorded by
    A. observing motor behavior responses closely
    B. observing paper-and-pencil performance in a group
    C. receiving information offered by parents
    D. receiving information offered by teachers

438. A therapist can best evaluate a child's social interaction skills by
    A. observing motor behavior responses closely
    B. observing the child in a group situation
    C. receiving information offered by parents
    D. receiving information offered by teachers

439. A 7-year-old child referred to occupational therapy was tested and evaluated and found to have eye-hand coordination problems, tactile and vestibular problems, social immaturity, and some visual perception and other sensory processing problems. The school reported some mild academic difficulties. The therapist stated that the child had
   A. a sensory integrative disorder called developmental dyspraxia
   B. a sensory integrative disorder called dysarthria
   C. a mild form of childhood neurosis
   D. a mild form of hyporeflexive postrotatory nystagmus

440. A 7-year-old child referred to occupational therapy because of difficulty in reading used each hand ipsilaterally. The therapist started evaluating for dysfunction in which area?
   A. Cognitive
   B. Sensory integration
   C. Motor planning
   D. Apathy

441. The Neonatal Behavioral Assessment Scale (NBAS) is well respected by pediatricians. This test assesses the infant's early
   A. reactions with overall behavior
   B. reactions with things in the environment
   C. behavior with the mother
   D. behavior and interaction with both animate and inanimate stimuli

442. The Neonatal Behavioral Assessment Scale is an assessment tool. To administer the tool, a therapist must
   A. have extensive experience with neonates and take specified training
   B. have extensive experience with neonates and be an OTR
   C. be an OTR and work in a neonatal facility
   D. complete the Ayres battery and many other tests prior to qualifying for the NBAS

QUESTIONS 443–446: In the evaluation of people with psychosocial dysfunction different group goals may be accomplished depending upon the type of group model used. Match the type of group with the group goals suggested below.

A. Activity group
B. Intrapsychic group
C. Social systems group
D. Growth group

443. Group goal focusing on the how of group behavior in the present.
444. Group goal attempting to achieve personality change through insight, tension reduction, and transference.
445. Group goal relating to the acquisition and maintenance of occupational performance.
446. Group goal attempting to increase a member's sensitivity to self and to others.

QUESTIONS 447–472: Select the **one** most appropriate answer.

447. In using a social systems group for the evaluation of people with psychosocial dysfunctions the therapist-leader's role is critical. To maintain the group as a social systems group, the therapist-leader tries to keep the group members' attention focused
    A. on both the "how" and "why"
    B. only on the "how"
    C. only on the "why"
    D. on either the "how" or the "why"

448. The therapist asks a person to do a very simple task with few instructions. The therapist seems to be testing
    A. sensory impairment
    B. range of motion
    C. cognition
    D. endurance

449. The therapist asks a person to do a very simple task that was completed the day before. The therapist seems to be testing
   A. sensory impairment
   B. range of motion
   C. cognition
   D. endurance

450. The therapist asks a person to pay attention to the task the therapist has assigned. The therapist seems to be testing
   A. sensory impairment
   B. range of motion
   C. cognition
   D. endurance

451. The therapist asks a person to do three or four things in a row. The therapist seems to be testing
   A. sensory impairment
   B. range of motion
   C. cognition
   D. endurance

452. The therapist tells a person to do the following: pinch the pinch gauge, lay it down, read the dial, and pick it up. The therapist seems to be testing
   A. hand strength
   B. range of motion
   C. cognition
   D. endurance

453. The therapist asks a person to talk about his/her daily routine, taking note of the amount of time and work needed to do a task and inquiring about the work output. The therapist seems to be testing
   A. hand strength
   B. range of motion
   C. cognition
   D. endurance

454. The therapist asks a person to put a simple jigsaw puzzle together that the person has completed and been timed for before. The therapist seems to be testing
    A. hand strength
    B. range of motion
    C. cognition
    D. endurance

455. The therapist instructs the patient to pick up different things around the department, some in warm sunlight, and then asks how the items feel. The therapist seems to be testing
    A. hand strength
    B. sensory impairment
    C. cognition
    D. endurance

456. The therapist asks a person to pick up a large variety of items and put them down and pick them up and put them down again. The therapist seems to be testing
    A. hand strength
    B. sensory impairment
    C. cognition
    D. endurance

457. The therapist places five small familiar object separately in the palm of a person's hand and makes sure the person has contact with the items with the thumb and the fingers. The therapist takes the items away and then asks the person to name all five items in order. The therapist seems to be testing
    A. hand strength
    B. sensory impairment
    C. cognition
    D. endurance

458. The Purdue Pegboard is most often used by therapists to evaluate
  A. gross movements of arms, hands, and fingers and fingertip dexterity
  B. hands and fingers and fingertip dexterity
  C. finger and fingertip dexterity only
  D. the speed and accuracy of the individual doing the task

459. The Bayley Scale of Infant Development is most often used by therapists to evaluate
  A. finger dexterity and gross motor movements
  B. gross motor movements only
  C. mental, motor, and behavioral ratings
  D. motor and behavioral ratings only

460. The Gesell Developmental Tests for age levels 5 to 10 are used by therapists to evaluate
  A. developmental growth
  B. mental growth for school readiness
  C. motor and adaptive skills
  D. IQ only

461. The Denver Developmental Screening Test is used by many therapists to evaluate
  A. development growth
  B. developmental delays
  C. IQ only
  D. reading ability

462. The Developmental Test of Visual-Motor Integration is used by many therapists to detect children with problems in visual-motor integration. The therapist administers this test to
  A. both individuals and groups
  B. only one individual at a time
  C. groups only
  D. boys or girls separately

463. The Marianne Frostig Developmental Test of Visual Perception is used by many therapists to detect children with problems in visual-motor integration. The therapist administers this test to
    A. both individuals and groups
    B. only one individual at a time
    C. groups only
    D. boys or girls separately

464. In the assessment of mildly, moderately, and even severely retarded persons, it is found that to questions about attitudes, abilities, and needs
    A. individuals can respond in a meaningful way
    B. individuals cannot respond in a meaningful way
    C. only certain of these groups can respond
    D. none of these groups can respond in a meaningful way

465. The therapist might use the Goodenough-Harris Drawing Test to
    A. establish a person's artistic ability
    B. determine a person's eye-hand coordination
    C. establish an appraisal of a person's personality
    D. determine a person's conceptual and intellectual maturity

466. The BaFPE (Bay Area Functional Performance) is used to
    A. measure some of the functions people must be able to perform in general activities of daily living
    B. determine the functions of people in group settings
    C. measure functional ability in one-on-one settings
    D. determine ability to act on the environment in specific goal-oriented ways

467. The Minnesota Multiphasic Personality Inventory (MMPI) is used by therapists to
    A. test the degree of emotional dysfunction
    B. determine IQ
    C. test the degree of personality dynamics
    D. determine PQ (personality quotient)

468. In the Signe Brunnstrom approach to hemiplegia, an evaluation is done to
   A. identify primitive spinal or brain stem postural reflexes and associated reactions
   B. identify upper and lower extremity synergy patterns and their associated reactions
   C. identify the proprioceptive neuromuscular facilitation (PNF) of maximal resistance in spiral and diagonal patterns of movement
   D. identify the reflex activity that dominates early motor behavior, which in turn reinforces the postural reflexes that support balance

469. The techniques of PNF were developed by
   A. Signe Brunnstrom, P.T.
   B. Herman Kabat, M.D.
   C. Margaret Knot, P.T.
   D. Dorothy Voss, P.T.

470. Assessment of motor function is necessary before treatment goals can be formulated and procedures and techniques selected. A sensory evaluation in the area of vision is made by the therapist to determine if the
   A. person has a normal range of vision
   B. eyes are infected and/or if the person needs glasses
   C. eyes move in all directions and the hands reach out
   D. eyes follow an object and lead the head in that direction

471. In a hand evaluation the therapist often measures the strength of the pinch using a pinch meter. Which of the following describes the tip pinch?
   A. The person pinches the meter between the pad of the thumb and the pads of the index and middle fingers
   B. The person pinches the meter between the pad of the thumb and the lateral surface of the index finger
   C. The person pinches the ends of the pinch meter between the tip of the pads of the thumb and the tip ends of the index and middle fingers
   D. The person pinches the ends of the pinch meter between the tip of the pads of the thumb and the tip ends of the middle and ring fingers

472. Which describes the palmar pinch?
   A. The person pinches the meter between the pad of the thumb and the pads of the index and middle fingers
   B. The person pinches the meter between the pads of the thumb and the pads of the palmar surface of the hand
   C. The person pinches the meter between the pad of the thumb and the palmar surface of the index finger
   D. The person pinches the meter between the palmar surface of the thumb and the pad of the index finger

QUESTIONS 473–476: Psychiatric occupational therapy is assessed or evaluated in several ways. Match the standard assessment tools (numbered) used by the therapist with the most appropriate evaluation procedure (lettered).

473. Observation
474. Interview
475. Data from other sources
476. Activity evaluation

A. A person shares information about his or her problems
B. A person has a careful identification of her or his skills recorded
C. Care is taken so that unnecessary duplication of effort does not take place
D. Notice that a person's place in the total group is consistently different

QUESTIONS 477–487: Select the one most appropriate answer.

477. One subtest of the BaFPE is the Task Oriented Assessment (TOA), which in turn uses five tasks. One task, "Sorting Skills," gives the therapist an evaluation of which of the primary perceptual-motor functions predominantly found in this task?
   A. Evidence of acalculia
   B. Evidence of bilateral integration
   C. Evidence of visual perception
   D. Evidence of agraphia

478. Another task of the BaFPE TOA is the "House Floor Plan." This task gives the therapist an evaluation of which of the primary perceptual-motor functions predominantly found in this task?
    A. Evidence of acalculia
    B. Evidence of bilateral integration
    C. Evidence of visual acuity
    D. Evidence of agraphia

479. Another task of the BaFPE TOA is the "Block Design." This task gives the therapist an evaluation of which of the primary perceptual-motor functions predominantly found in this task?
    A. Evidence of acalculia
    B. Evidence of bilateral integration
    C. Evidence of visual perception
    D. Evidence of agraphia

480. The other subtest of the BaFPE is the Social Interaction Scale (SIS). This subtest gives the therapist an evaluation of which of the following in working with a person with psychiatric dysfunction?
    A. some of the functions people must be able to perform in general activities of daily living
    B. the behavior of an individual in a social situation
    C. a group of people in a psychiatric occupational therapy department
    D. the presence or absence of certain observable aspects of behavior

481. The tone of the process of assessment is one that should lead directly to the establishment of objectives for a given person's treatment. Overall objectives are usually developed by
    A. the occupational therapist assigned to that person
    B. the occupational therapy staff responsible for the service
    C. the team assigned to the person in treatment
    D. the psychiatrist assigned to that person

482. In evaluation for occupational therapy treatment it is necessary to
    A. start treatment as soon as the client arrives
    B. get the client diagnosis and start from there
    C. collect and organize relevant data before seeing the client
    D. rely on past experience as it is the best judge of effective treatment

483. If in an evaluation, the stretch reflex is found to be abnormal throughout the body, all of the reflexes will be
    A. abnormal
    B. normal
    C. asymmetrical
    D. symmetrical

484. If in an evaluation, the stretch reflex is found to be abnormal in only part of the body, the related reflexes will be
    A. abnormal
    B. normal
    C. asymmetrical
    D. symmetrical

485. Tonic reflexes that govern the distribution of muscle tone throughout the body are most obvious at specific ages during infancy. They remain with us
    A. through infancy
    B. throughout life
    C. only in times of stress
    D. only in times of fatigue

486. It is possible to use reflexes to determine the chronological age of premature infants. In an evaluation of gestational age a more accurate assessment would be
    A. comparison of development with normal infant charts
    B. comparison of development with other atypical infant charts
    C. combination of an evaluation of neurological signs with external physical characteristics
    D. combination of an evaluation of normal developmental sequences with a chart on reflex development

487. Resting postures are basically a reflection on the background muscle tone present in an infant at rest. An experienced therapist can assess muscle tone by
    A. looking at an infant's postures
    B. picking up the sleeping infant and recording its reactions
    C. recording reactions upon waking the infant
    D. rolling the infant over, holding the head in midline

QUESTIONS 488–491: In the assessment of a client for prevocational and vocational evaluation, a number of commercial systems are available. Match the system with the assessment tools most commonly used in that system.

   A. Occupational clusters of related jobs
   B. Work sample recordings
   C. Psychological tests and ratings
   D. Eight accepted instruments based on five neuropsychological factors

488. The Hester Evaluation System
489. The McCarron-Dial Work Evaluation Series
490. The Philadelphia Jewish Employment and Vocational System
491. The Talent Assessment Program

QUESTIONS 492–499: Select the **one** most appropriate answer.

492. In the evaluation of clients with problems of addiction, the question of the need for perceptual or sensory integrative dysfunction assessment is based upon
    A. a low level of self-esteem
    B. a regression to oral levels of emotional need
    C. underlying depression and limited coping strategies
    D. a deficit in an ability to process information

493. In the assessment of a hospitalized person with chronic schizophrenia who is regressed and withdrawn, the most likely place to start would be
    A. the development of adaptive habit patterns
    B. administration of a formal assessment battery
    C. collection of data from observations, family, and peers
    D. planning of a safe environment with a high level of interaction

494. In the assessment of a delinquent adolescent faced with possible punishment, the therapist should try and develop an atmosphere of
    A. discipline
    B. trust
    C. learning
    D. confrontation

495. The assessment process should be viewed as an attempt by the therapist to collaborate with an anorexic adolescent in
    A. identifying situations in which the adolescent has typically felt out of control or incompetent
    B. identifying the pattern of eating and the amount
    C. identifying an occupational choice and pursuing its development
    D. identifying the nutritional value of foods for a proper diet

496. Because of the extreme sense of hopelessness and doom experienced by the depressed person, engaging the individual in the evaluation process is
    A. easy, as the person can only go up and needs company
    B. difficult, as the person states he or she has no interests and wants to be left alone
    C. random, as the person has had past experiences and one good experience can be found
    D. scientific, as more people in the United States seek mental health services for depression than any other problem

497. One of the newer roles and focuses of treatment for occupational therapists has been elaborated and defined by Gary Kielhofner. From his perspective therapists would describe their work as
   A. evaluation of a client from the etiology and prognosis
   B. evaluation of activities as they relate to pathological dynamics
   C. evaluation of a client's dynamics as they relate to an activity analysis
   D. evaluation of a client's occupational nature and the dynamics of occupational dysfunction

498. In the evaluation of a person to determine the difference between mild and profound retardation, the many instruments available can be used
   A. with little or no problem
   B. with ease for efficiency in content
   C. with ease for efficiency in format
   D. with difficulty, as most instruments cannot span this distance effectively

499. There are a number of approaches to assessment of occupational function in mentally retarded persons. One of the least commonly accepted and used of these approaches is
   A. direct testing of criterion behaviors in real or simulated settings
   B. observations accompanies by a rating scale of behavior
   C. knowledge measurements conducted with competent measurement tools
   D. individual competencies evaluated against criteria required by the environment of concern

Explanatory Answers

400. (C) Self-maintenance is evaluated in terms of activities needed to maintain an individual's life support needs and his/her ability and skill to fulfill these needs (e.g., dressing, toileting, eating, and mobility). (REF. 18, p. 12)

401. (B) Productivity is evaluated in terms of a person's skill in certain work settings, punctuality, and ability to follow directions and use judgment. (REF. 18, p. 12)

402. (A) Leisure is evaluated by examining the types of activities in which a person participates for individual enjoyment. (REF. 18, p. 13)

403. (C) The motor component of performance is evaluated to see if the patient's neuromuscular/skeletal system is able to perform the basic movement required for occupational therapy. (REF. 18, p. 13)

404. (B) A sensory component of performance is evaluated to determine if the senses are able to function separately and together and with the motor component to permit efficient body activity. (REF. 18, p. 13)

405. (C) A cognitive component of performance is evaluated to see if the patient can attend to a task in order to learn it and perform it, solve problems, and remember information and skills over short and long periods of time. (REF. 18, p. 13)

406. (A) An intrapersonal component of performance is evaluated to establish a patient's ability to distinguish reality from unreality and to be able to deal with reality. (REF. 18, p. 13)

407. (A) An interpersonal component of performance is evaluated to see how well a person is able to relate and to get along with other people. (REF. 18, p. 13)

408. (C) Normal and above-normal performance skills are often overlooked in evaluation; yet these may be the most useful ones in developing and restoring skills as well as in recognizing dysfunctions. (REF. 18, p. 81)

409. (B) The primary purposes of an evaluation are to gather, analyze, and interpret data so treatment can start or other dispositions can take place. (REF. 18, p. 83)

410. (A) Prior to an evaluation a disadvantage might be to look only for those behaviors reported, while an advantage might be to compare what has been reported with direct observations to come up with an honest assessment. (REF. 17, p. 165)

411. (B) Through a study of the child's history, the therapist is guided by which evaluation process to use prior to knowing the child's dysfunction, planning for treatment, or even consulting the physician. (REF. 17, p. 165)

412. (B) An evaluation is chosen that incorporates 2- to 3-year-old tasks with a few additional tasks at both extremes to include behavior not noted in the history. (REF. 17, p. 165)

413. (C) When the unexpected is expected, the therapist can function more confidently and more responsibly than would be possible if he/she were not mentally prepared for whatever might occur. (REF. 17, p. 165)

414. (D) No matter what the content of the interview, the prime objective is to show the family members that the therapist is genuinely interested in their problem and is ready to listen to their story. (REF. 17, p. 167)

415. (C) Each treatment session should be assessed and each target area reviewed to determine the effectiveness of the activity practice and to revise the objectives as they are mastered or found to be unreachable. This function is not a research process unless it is detailed in a research design, and patients may or may not be aware of the therapist's ability. (REF. 15, p. 143)

Evaluation / 111

416. (D) A therapist must meet two essential requirements to conduct a successful interview: (1) a solid knowledge base must underlie the therapist's selection of questions or areas to be covered and (2) skills in active listening must exist in order to play a vital involved role demonstrating respect for the patient. (REF. 15, p. 145)

417. (D) Manual muscle testing is rated by having a patient move a body part through its full ROM first against gravity and then against gravity and resistance. (REF. 15, p. 149)

418. (C) A rating of F (Fair) or 3 is a complete ROM against gravity; with gravity eliminated it is P (Poor) or 2; against gravity with full resistance it is N (Normal) or 5; and with some resistance it is G (Good) or 4. (REF. 15, p. 149)

419. (A) To maintain reliability and accuracy each time a patient is evaluated for ROM, the same therapist should measure the patient using the same method at the same time of day. (REF. 15, p. 149)

420. (B) When an evaluation of a patient with a central nervous system dysfunction is expected, consideration needs to be given to all influences on coordinated voluntary control of movement. Evaluation of the dysfunctions depends upon the obvious problems that seem to exist relative to the dysfunction. (REF. 16, p. 46)

421. (B) Passive movement of an extremity is used to evaluate muscle tone. (REF. 16, p. 47)

422. (C) If muscle tone is increased, there will be an increased resistance to passive movement. (REF. 16, p. 47)

423. (A) A reflex is an involuntary, stereotyped response to a particular stimulus developed in fetal life and continues to dominate motor behavior through early infancy. (REF. 16, p. 48)

424. (D) Neither a positive nor a negative response can be equated with normal without considering whether a positive or negative response is normal for the age range. **(REF. 16, p. 49)**

425. (C) Pressure to the palm of the hand on the ulnar side results in a grasp reflex in a child from birth to 3 or 4 months of age. **(REF. 16, p. 50)**

426. (C) Uncontrolled flexion of the leg is the result of application of a quick tactile stimulus to the sole of one foot in a normal child from birth to 2 months. **(REF. 16, p. 50)**

427. (D) Uncontrolled extension of a leg that has been stimulated occurs when pressure is applied to the ball of the foot of that flexed leg in a child from birth to 2 months old put into the supine position, head in midline, with one leg extended and the other fully flexed. **(REF. 16, p. 50)**

428. (A) Extension of the leg opposite to the one stimulated with hip adduction and internal rotation is the response to a passively flexed extended leg of an infant who is in the supine position, head in midline, with one leg extended and the stimulated leg fully flexed. **(REF. 16, p. 50)**

429. (B) Hip adduction and internal rotation of the opposite leg are the responses to the stimulus of tapping the adductor surface of the thigh in an infant who is supine, with head in midline and both legs extended, and has hip flexor tightness of spasticity. **(REF. 16, p. 50)**

430. (D) Extension of the limbs on the face side and flexion of the limbs on the skull side are the responses to an asymmetrical tonic neck reflex in a child from birth to 4 months. **(REF. 16, p. 50)**

431. (D) The stimulus of placing a normal child from birth to 4 months of age in the prone position with the head in the midline position results in flexion of the extremities or increased flexor tone in the extremities. No other stimulus is needed. (REF. 16, p. 51)

432. (B) The body of a child will rotate as a whole in the direction to which the head is turned if placed in a supine position with the arms and legs extended. (REF. 16, p. 51)

433. (C) The body-righting activity of a normal child of 6 months to 5 years who is in the supine position with arms and legs extended and the head turned to one side is that the body will rotate around its axis, in the same direction, so that it starts at the shoulder, then the trunk, and then the pelvis. (REF. 16, p. 51)

434. (B) To obtain valid results on a standardized test, the therapist must follow the procedures stipulated by the author for the presentation of the test. (REF. 17, p. 175)

435. (B) To obtain valid results on a standardized test, the therapist must follow the procedures stipulated by the author for scoring and/or analyzing the test results. (REF. 17, p. 175)

436. (D) Some tests used in occupational therapy require that the examiners receive special training and certification before they are allowed to administer them. (REF. 17, p. 175)

437. (A) Sensory integrative and motor functions can be observed by closely evaluating a child's motor behavior. (REF. 17, p. 175)

438. (B) Group evaluation by the therapist is appropriate for assessing a child's social interaction skills. (REF. 17, p. 175)

439. (A) A sensory integrative disorder called developmental dyspraxia is a disorder of motor planning wherein tactile and vestibular system problems appear to contribute to motor planning and make it difficult to perform eye-hand functions. All problems seem to contribute to social and academic difficulties. (REF. 17, p. 248)

440. (B) Individuals with sensory integrative dysfunctions often show a marked inability to read or use both hands together, and it is hypothesized that these symptoms involve deficiencies in interhemispheral communication. (REF. 17, p. 249)

441. (D) The NBAS assesses the infant's early behavior and interaction with both animate and inanimate environmental stimuli. (REF. 17, p. 251)

442. (A) To qualify to administer the NBAS a therapist must have had experience with neonates, received special training, administered the test 12-15 times, taken training sessions, and had annual follow-up checkouts. (REF. 17, p. 252)

443. (C) A social systems group is the type of group used to focus on the how of group behavior in the present. (REF. 28, p. 26)

444. (B) An intrapsychic group is used to achieve personality change through insight, tension reduction, and the use of transference. (REF. 28, p. 26)

445. (A) An activity group is used as it is related to the acquisition and maintenance of occupational performance. (REF. 28, p. 26)

446. (D) A growth group is used to increase a member's sensitivity to self and to others. (REF. 28, p. 26)

447. (B) In using a social systems group the leader tries to keep the member's attention focused on the "how" rather than the "why" or on the here and now events. Focusing on the "why" leads into intrapsychic issues and to a different type of group. (REF. 28, p. 31)

448. (C) The therapist is testing for cognition, which is made up
449. (C) of some of, but is not limited to, the following: ability
450. (C) to follow simple instructions, ability to carry over
451. (C) learned skills from one day to the next, ability to attend
452. (C) to a task or check on attention span, ability to follow numerous steps in a process, and ability to perform in a logical sequence. (REF. 15, p. 153)

453. (D) A person is often tested for ability to reach or maintain the necessary energy output required to do certain things. The therapist will carefully keep track of the amount of work and time required to do it and also the output from the work. This is part of testing the person's endurance. (REF. 15, p. 153)

454. (C) The therapist is testing for cognition when trying to determine if a person can perform a task by organizing parts into a meaningful whole. (REF. 15, p. 153)

455. (B) The therapist is testing for sensory impairment (temperature) when the patient is instructed to pick up items that are warm or at room temperature and say how they feel. If all the items were at room temperature the therapist might be testing tactile sense. (REF. 15, p. 153)

456. (B) The therapist is testing for sensory impairment (proprioception) by having the person move his arms up and down a number of times. (REF. 15, p. 153)

457. (C) The therapist is testing for cognition by testing a person's ability to concentrate and recall the items placed in the hand. If each object were only to be identified, the therapist would be testing for stereognosis. (REF. 15, p. 153)

458. (A) The Purdue Pegboard measures for gross movements of arms, hands, and fingers and fingertip dexterity. (REF. 15, p. 167)

459. (A) The Bayley Scale provides mental, motor, and behavior ratings for ages 2 to 30 months. (REF. 15, p. 159)

460. (B) The Gesell Developmental Tests rate mental growth to aid in determining school readiness. (REF. 15, p. 160)

461. (B) The Denver Test is used to screen infants and children for developmental delays. Areas evaluated are gross motor, fine motor, language, and personal-social development for ages 2 weeks to 6 years 3 months. (REF. 15, p. 169)

462. (A) The Developmental Test of Visual-Motor Integration can be administered to groups. Emphasis is on preschool groups. It has long and short forms and separate norms for each sex. (REF. 15, p. 160)

463. (A) The Marianne Frostig Test has five subtests and can be administered to individuals and groups. (REF. 15, p. 161)

464. (A) A number of studies with mildly, moderately, and even severely retarded persons have supported the belief that retarded individuals can respond in a meaningful way to questions about their attitudes, abilities, and needs. (REF. 20, p. 384)

465. (D) The Goodenough-Harris Drawing Test is designed to test the accuracy of observations and the development of conceptual thinking and, hence, conceptual and intellectual thinking. (REF. 15, p. 163)

466. (A) The BaFPE is designed to assess in a consistent and measurable way some of the functions that people must be able to perform in general acitivities of daily living. It is made up of two subtests: one measures general ability to act on the environment in specific goal-oriented ways and the other assesses general ability to relate appropriately to other people. (REF. 27, p. 255)

467. (A) The MMPI assesses the type and degree of emotional dysfunction in adults (REF. 15, p. 164)

468. (A) The Signe Brunnstrom evaluation of hemiplegia is done to identify primitive spinal or brain stem postural reflexes and associated reactions and also the stage of recovery of voluntary control of movement and sensory disturbances. (REF. 16, p. 97)

469. (B) Herman Kabat developed the techniques of PNF. (REF. 16, p. 106)

470. (D) Vision is evaluated to determine if the eyes follow an object and lead the movement of the head. (REF. 16, p. 109)

471. (C) The tip pinch is measured by pinching the ends of the pinch meter between the tip of the pad of the thumb and the tip ends of the index and middle fingers. (REF. 16, p. 226)

472. (A) The palmar pinch is measured by pinching the meter between the pad of the thumb and the pads of the index and middle fingers. (REF. 16, p. 226)

473. (D) The skill of the therapist to observe well is critical to all kinds of assessment procedures. Observing a group activity and noticing a person consistently sitting outside of the main circle means something. (REF. 15, p. 304)

474. (A) An interview is a planned conversation conducted for a specific purpose. In such an interview the person with a problem has an opportunity to share information about the problem. (REF. 15, p. 304)

475. (C) There is a wealth of information available from other team members when they work together. Working and communicating together will prevent unnecessary duplication of effort. (REF. 15, p. 305)

476. (B) The careful identification of skills required to carry out activities is the key to treatment in occupational therapy as a whole. (REF. 15, p. 305)

477. (B) The "Sorting Skills" subtask of the BaFPE TOA provides the therapist with an evaluation of possible evidence of bilateral integration; ability to cross the midline; size, shape, and color discrimination, and motor apraxia, to name a few. (REF. 27, p. 269)

478. (D) The "House Floor Plan" subtask of the BaFPE TOA provides the therapist with an evaluation of possible evidence of agraphia, visual perception, logical proportion, judgment related to spatial relationships, and abstraction, to name a few. (REF. 27, p. 269)

479. (C) The "Block Design" subtask of the BaFPE TOA provides the therapist with an evaluation of possible evidence of visual perception, short-term memory, more accuracy, figure/ground perception, and discrimination, to name a few. (REF. 27, p. 269)

480. (B) The SIS subtest allows the therapist to assess the behavior of an individual with a psychiatric dysfunction in a social situation. The subtest is for individuals versus groups and uses a rating scale rather than a checklist, as a rating scale defines a continuum of dimensions while a checklist reports only the presence or absence of certain behaviors. (REF. 27, p. 270)

481. (C) The tone of the process of assessment is one that should lead directly to the setting of objectives. Overall objectives are usually developed by the team assigned to that person. (REF. 15; p. 308)

482. (C) The evaluation process represents an organized and systematic way of determining the client's needs. It is essential to implementation, objective setting, and assessment of the effectiveness of the treatment plan. (REF. 15, p. 144)

483. (A) If the stretch reflex is abnormal throughout the body, all reflexes will be abnormal, as the stretch reflex contributes to muscle tone, which supports all movement. (REF. 15, p. 176)

484. (A) If the stretch reflex is abnormal in only part of the body the related reflexes will be abnormal, as the stretch reflex contributes to muscle tone throughout the body. (REF. 15, p. 176)

485. (B) Tonic reflexes are most obvious at specific ages during infancy but remain throughout life and are most evident at times of stress or fatigue. (REF. 15, p. 176)

486. (C) A more accurate assessment of gestational age results from combining the evaluation of neurological signs with external physical characteristics. A consistent rule in normal development is that there is no rule, and a glance at a reflex chart would reveal tremendous variations in reflex development. (REF. 15, p. 177)

487. (A) When an infant is sleeping, muscle tone falls so low as to approach flaccidity. An experienced therapist can assess the infant simply by looking at the infant's postures. A normal infant will have no single position dominating. (REF. 15, p. 178)

488. (C) The Hester Evaluation System is not a work sample system but a battery of psychological tests and ratings correlated with the Dictionary of Occupational Titles. (REF. 15, p. 210)

489. (D) This system involves eight widely accepted instruments based upon five neuropsychological factors. These instruments are primarily psychometric in nature. (REF. 14, p. 210)

490. (B) The Philadelphia Jewish Employment and Vocational System uses 28 work sample recording observations and feedback based upon the Worker Trait Group Organization of the Dictionary of Occupational Titles. (REF. 15, p. 210)

491. (A) The Talent Assessment Program is based on occupational clusters of related jobs and is geared to the assessment of perceptions and dexterities. (REF. 15, p. 211)

492. (D) In observations of clients with problems of addiction, there appears to be a deficit in their ability to process information from their environment. This together with an apparent need for intensity of experience raises the question of the need of a perceptual or sensory integrative evaluation. (REF. 15, p. 324)

493. (C) A hospitalized person with chronic schizophrenia who is withdrawn and regressed should be evaluated by collecting data from observation, family, and peers, because an assessment battery would overwhelm the person as would a high level of interaction. (REF. 20, p. 294)

494. (B) The delinquent adolescent faced with possible punishment for behavior may pose a difficult problem for obtaining reliable and valid data. Therefore, an assessment should proceed in an atmosphere of trust in which a nonjudgmental, open, exploratory attitude is maintained. (REF. 20, p. 285)

495. **(A)** A key issue for the anorexic person may be his/her feelings of being manipulated or controlled by others. Therefore, the occupational therapist should attempt to identify these situations and develop situations that contradict these feelings of inefficacy. (REF. 20, p. 276)

496. **(B)** Because the depressed person experiences a sense of hopelessness and doom and states he or she has no interests and no future and want to be left alone, the evaluation process is quite difficult. (REF. 20, p. 265)

497. **(D)** Gary Kielhofner has written extensively on a model that begins by looking at the occupational nature of persons. The model of human occupations is used to explore the dynamics of occupational dysfunction. (REF. 20, p. 248)

498. **(D)** There are extreme differences in typical behavior between mildly and profoundly retarded persons. Many instruments cannot span this distance effectively in terms of either content or format. Therefore, most instruments can be used most appropriately for only part of this continuum. (REF. 20, p. 383)

499. **(C)** Knowledge measurements for the assessment of occupational function in the mentally retarded constitute the least commonly used and accepted method of evaluation. (REF. 20, 9. 303)

7 Planning

QUESTIONS 500–536: Select the **one** most appropriate answer.

500. In planning for the use of an activity the therapist should assume that
    A. since everyone participates in activities, the patient also should be involved in them
    B. activities have a role to play in the development of a physically sound and well-integrated personality
    C. activities are an easy way to treat different dysfunctions
    D. occupational therapy is based on activity and, therefore, activities should be used

501. A therapist can further assume in planning the use of an activity that a person might be able to
    A. learn a new occupation
    B. learn a better way to utilize time
    C. attain a sense of mastery and well-being in the process
    D. attain a way of making extra money while at home or at the hospital

502. In utilizing activities in planning programs therapists may assume that activities
    A. are universally used by all therapists
    B. are regulated by skills learned in school
    C. are socioculturally regulated by values and beliefs
    D. have little or no extrinsic value and thus can be used any way one wishes

503. In planning an activity for a person in a certain age group the therapist should be aware that
    A. activity related to age varies from society to society
    B. the person has the physical capacity to perform the activity
    C. others of the same age in the service area are doing the activity
    D. the activity is highly successful for the person's dysfunction and thus overrides other considerations

504. In planning an activity for a person of a certain sex the therapist should be aware that
    A. activity related to sex varies from society to society
    B. activity related to sex varies little from society to society
    C. others of the same sex should be in the service area when activity is instigated
    D. the activity is highly successful for the person's dysfunction and thus overrides other considerations

505. In planning group activities for young people from the same age and background and mixed sexes the therapist, cognizant of sex-role blurring in today's service areas, can plan
    A. the same activities for both sexes
    B. different activities for each sex group
    C. a different activity for each person in the group
    D. the schedule so that each sex group arrives at different times

506. In planning activities the therapist can make the assumption about humankind that
   A. people are different and no one assumption can be made
   B. individuals who are sick do not wish to change
   C. individuals can change and indeed desire change
   D. all people who are sick wish others to make changes for them

507. In planning an activity such as eating a therapist needs to be aware that this activity
   A. is a single universal category
   B. may fit into more than one category
   C. need not be considered as belonging in any category
   D. is good for any person at any time because everyone has to eat

508. In planning an activity the therapist should consider the notion of activities in a field of action so that the activity
   A. is interesting and exciting to the patient
   B. is interesting and exciting to those around the patient
   C. simulates as nearly as possible the action of others
   D. simulates as nearly as possible conditions in the real world

509. In planning an activity in a field of action a therapist follows rules governed by the conduct of the specific activity. These rules are
   A. implicit -- ingrained from past experiences and automatic
   B. explicit -- specific directives that are communicated verbally
   C. both implicit and explicit
   D. really of little value because each service area has its own rules that supersede other outside rules

510. In planning an activity a therapist should keep in mind that to help a person achieve a sense of accomplishment or competence
    A. a task needs a beginning and an end
    B. the time factor for a task is unimportant because success in doing a part is enough
    C. a task has to be liked to be successful
    D. a task has to create interest in those around the person to be successful

511. An activity that is "approved" or appropriate for a given age group, class, and sex will give the therapist an advantage in planning if the activity
    A. requires skill that is a little beyond that now possessed by the person
    B. requires no more skill than that possessed by the person
    C. requires barely any skill at all
    D. does not require that skill be a component of the planning process

512. In planning a treatment program the therapist, in using herself or himself as well as an activity, should keep in mind that in a day-to-day situation the therapist should present a model for the person to
    A. imitate
    B. interact with
    C, like
    D. respect

513. In planning an activity a therapist should remember that activities are therapeutic when they enable change to take place
    A. in all patients with equal success
    B. in some patients with equal success
    C. in any direction with any dysfunction
    D. in a direction from dysfunction to function

514. In planning activities that are therapeutic the therapist should remember that activities will enable change to take place if they have
   A. meaning and relevance to the individual
   B. proven meaning and relevance to entire groups
   C. meaning to the individual
   D. relevance only to the individual

515. In planning activities to enable change to occur the therapist should remember that activities must be systematically organized and administered according to principles derived from
   A. the concept "if it works use it"
   B. the concept that "what works for one will work for another"
   C. an approach based on a theoretical rationale
   D. an approach based on data provided by your school

516. In planning activities for a patient the therapist should
   A. use an intuitive approach based upon years of experience
   B. use or develop an activity inventory showing a chronological listing of the person's past activities
   C. shy away from past experience because the person's current level is where to start
   D. try the person out on a number of different activities to see which ones seem to work best

517. In planning a therapeutic program, establishing goals that meet the person's needs is of primary concern. The next most likely concern would be to see if
   A. the attending physician approves of the goals
   B. the occupational therapy supervisor approves of the goals
   C. goals can be carried out within the constraints of the therapeutic situation
   D. the family can afford the time it takes to meet the goals

518. In planning both long-range overall goals and short-term goals the therapist should be aware that
    A. each set of goals is completely separated by a time frame
    B. at times both sets of goals may merge
    C. the person may not wish you to plan long-range goals
    D. the physician may not want you to plan long-range goals

519. After an evaluation process and in the planning stages the therapist (to effect maximal function) should
    A. use the simplest and least amount of equipment
    B. use a lot of equipment to check everything out
    C. use equipment only after the person has tried and cannot complete a function
    D. not use any equipment until the person feels secure and comfortable in the service area

520. In planning, the therapist should schedule activities so that there is sufficient frequency of repetition and duration to
    A. have the person feel secure and comfortable in the service area
    B. have the person become familiar with routine
    C. ensure an integration of learning
    D. assure the person, family, and physician that everything planned will be accomplished

521. In planning activities the therapist (to ensure adequate evaluation) should
    A. schedule more time than needed to do an occasional evaluation
    B. schedule evaluations of progress at specific times
    C. schedule evaluations when progress is noted
    D. schedule times for evaluations prior to staffing and discharge

522. In planning a program for persons over 65 years who have experienced physical decline and require more energy to care for and maintain their bodies, it would be expected that part of the therapist's job in helping people return to their own homes is
 A. explaining that a great deal of independence must be relinquished
 B. explaining that Social Security and its new dimensions will take care of new problems encountered
 C. explaining that everyone else in that age group is in the same situation so that learning to cope will not be a problem
 D. explaining that working hard in occupational therapy will overcome most handicaps and that readjusting to the previous lifestyle will be no problem

523. When dealing with an older person in planning any activity, the therapist needs to be aware that more energy is needed and
 A. some new patterns of life need to be initiated
 B. old patterns can be kept if proper timing is used
 C. the correct activities will help maintain proper levels of energy
 D. the correct activities will generate enough energy

524. In planning for an older person the therapist needs to be aware that as the person's social world begins to diminish
 A. more activities need to be planned to fill the gap
 B. fewer activities are needed in keeping with the diminished social life
 C. loneliness often becomes an established consequence
 D. community agencies have been developed to take the place of the person's former social world

525. In the planning process for the geriatric population the geriatric specialist or therapist should be aware of and knowledgeable about the latest legislative programs offered to older persons, because this will enable therapists to
   A. discuss these programs intelligently
   B. inform persons in need of programs about what is available
   C. make sure others on the team know about new programs
   D. inform persons in need of programs where to go if they are not receiving proper care

526. In planning a treatment program for older people the therapist should be aware that very often
   A. two chronic diseases may be involved simultaneously in one person
   B. usually only one chronic disease affects a person at a time
   C. if two chronic diseases are present, one takes a major role and the other takes a minor role
   D. only one chronic disease can be worked on at one time

527. In planning a program for a person with more than one chronic disease it is paramount that the therapist
   A. acquire a firm knowledge of the diseases prevalent among older people
   B. acquire a firm knowledge of one or two diseases and check on others as needed
   C. know where to find additional information when necessary
   D. be aware of who on the team knows about a specific disease in order to check with them

528. In planning an overall treatment program for someone who is in need of reinforced learning and needs to ameliorate disorientation and confusion a therapist will choose to schedule a person in
   A. a traditional activity program in occupational therapy
   B. an attitude therapy program
   C. a reality orientation program
   D. a remotivation program

529. In planning an overall treatment program for someone who is in need of reinforcing desirable behavior a therapist should schedule a person in
   A. a traditional activity program in occupational therapy
   B. an attitude therapy program
   C. a reality orientation program
   D. a remotivation program

530. In planning an overall treatment program for someone who is moderately confused and need to become more interested in their surroundings and environment a therapist should schedule a person in
   A. a traditional activity program in occupational therapy
   B. an attitude therapy program
   C. a reality orientation program
   D. a remotivation program

531. In planning an overall treatment program for a person, the therapist should be aware that a reality orientation program involves
   A. a formal setting, is focused on an individual, and is consistent every day until change occurs
   B. a semiformal setting, usually 5 to 12 people at a time, and one 30- to 60-minute session weekly for 12 weeks
   C. a formal setting and 4 to 5 people in a class, meeting 5 times per week until the class graduates
   D. a formal setting, is focused on one or more persons at a time, and lasts 30 to 60 minutes 5 times per week until change occurs

532. In planning an overall treatment program for a person the therapist should be aware that an attitude therapy program involves
   A. a formal setting, is focused on an individual, and is consistent every day until change occurs
   B. a semiformal setting, usually 5 to 12 people at a time, and one 30- to 60-minute session weekly for 12 weeks
   C. a formal setting and 4 to 5 people in a class, meeting 5 times per week until the class graduates
   D. a formal setting, is focused on one or more persons at a time, and lasts 30 to 60 minutes 5 times per week until change occurs

533. In planning an overall treatment program for a person the therapist should be aware that a remotivation program involves
   A. a formal setting, is focused on an individual, and is consistent every day until change occurs
   B. a semiformal setting, usually 5 to 12 people at a time, and one 30- to 60-minute session weekly for 12 weeks
   C. a formal setting and 4 to 5 people in a class, meeting 5 times per week until the class graduates
   D. a formal setting, is focused on one or more persons at a time, and lasts 30 to 60 minutes 5 times per week until change occurs

534. In planning a therapeutic craft program for a person, the therapist would do well to keep in mind that
   A. a therapeutic craft program is often misunderstood by the patient and other health professionals
   B. a therapeutic craft program no longer needs explanation because occupational therapy is over 60 years old
   C. therapeutic crafts are used by many kinds of therapists and others so misunderstanding is minimal
   D. today's OTR uses crafts infrequently and thus crafts should not be used if another activity can be found

535. In planning a hospital adjustment program for a terminally ill person, the therapist should keep in mind that as a result of modern technology, life expectancy is almost twice that of our ancestors. Because of this and other factors, our society tends to treat death as
    A. a remote possibility
    B. an immediate and perpetual menace
    C. something each of us must endure
    D. something that will be removed and/or postponed in the hospital

536. In planning on working with a terminally ill person a therapist should know that social scientists believe that the fear of death is universal. The therapist should further be aware that Americans generally seem to cope with death by
    A. making plans for their demise
    B. using avoidance, denial, and repudiation
    C. asking their family members to make plans for them
    D. using the time with a therapist to learn to accept death

132 / Occupational Therapy

QUESTIONS 537–539: In planning on working with terminally ill people a therapist should know that there are coping techniques and stages associated with death and dying. Match each worker with the group that describes his/her/their understanding of the death and dying process.

A.
1. Chronological age and distance from death
2. Physical and mental health
3. Various frames of reference
4. Community attitudes
5. Family and personal experiences related to death
6. Attitudes of people within the immediate environment
7. The individual's psychological maturity and integrity

B.
1. Denial
2. Anger
3. Bargaining
4. Organization and completion of unfinished business
5. Depression
6. Acceptance

C.
1. Repudiation of getting older
2. Denial of the extension of aging
3. Denial of irreversible decline
4. Impaired autonomy
5. A yielding of control and counter control
6. Cessation of life

D.
1. Planning the funeral arrangements
2. Writing the will and last testament
3. Bringing all insurance policies up to date
4. Purchasing the cemetery lot
5. Making peace with family members
6. Taking care that all the bills will be paid

537. Kubler-Ross
538. Jeffers and Verwoerdt
539. Weisman

QUESTIONS 540–555: Select the one most appropriate answer.

540. In planning to work with a terminally ill person a therapist should know that some professional teams agree that in the area of death and dying most health care professionals
   A. are very understanding of the death and dying process
   B. impose emotional isolation upon the dying person
   C. do not think the person will die
   D. do all they can to help the person enjoy the last days of life

541. In planning an activity designed to meet a goal of decreasing an undesirable behavior the therapist should
   A. always attempt to increase an acceptable behavior when trying to decrease an unacceptable one
   B. always attempt to increase acceptable behavior and know that unacceptable behavior will automatically decrease
   C. work on only one behavior at a time -- increase acceptable behavior and then work on decreasing unacceptable behavior
   D. work on only one behavior at a time -- decrease unacceptable behavior and then work on increasing acceptable behavior

542. In planning psychiatric treatment objectives and developing a mutual understanding on the part of the person for whom the objectives are planned the therapist should
   A. write them up and put them in file with a copy to the person involved
   B. develop them with the person for whom they are intended
   C. write them up and present them only to the team members for approval
   D. develop them and present them only to the psychiatrist in charge

543. In terms of the therapist who writes them, treatment plans represent, among other things,
    A. the therapist's compassion for people for whom they are assigned and responsible
    B. the therapist's complete understanding of other team members' contributions to the treatment process
    C. a synthesis of the therapist's knowledge of an activity and its relationship to growth and performance
    D. a synthesis of the therapist's ability to understand personal dynamics and their functions

544. Planning involves setting goals. The therapist should maintain the attitude that the determination of life goals should rest with
    A. the team, regardless of what the therapist agrees to
    B. the person involved, regardless of what the therapist or team agrees to
    C. the physician, regardless of what the therapist or team agrees to
    D. the family, regardless of what the staff agrees to

545. In planning a program the therapist becomes aware that the person for whom the program is planned does not respond readily to that program and that person's prognosis is poor. The therapist's attitude should be that
    A. other people need occupational therapy service more and plans for discontinuance should be started
    B. this person needs additional attention and should receive special time in occupational therapy
    C. this person and any other deserve the best occupational therapy that can be offered
    D. a person with that attitude and prognosis should be cared for by someone less skilled

546. In planning the transfer of a quadriplegic person who has weak elbow flexion and weak shoulder musculature, one should use a
    A. sliding transfer
    B. depression transfer
    C. pivot transfer
    D. lift (Hoyer or other brand name)

547. In planning the transfer of a quadriplegic person who is unable to move, one should use a
  A. sliding transfer
  B. depression transfer
  C. pivot transfer
  D. lift (Hoyer or other brand name)

548. In planning the transfer of a person who is unable to bear weight on the lower extremities, but has strong upper extremities, one should use a
  A. sliding transfer
  B. depression transfer
  C. pivot transfer
  D. lift (Hoyer or other brand name)

549. In planning the transfer of a person who has weight bearing on the lower extremities, one should use a
  A. sliding transfer
  B. depression transfer
  C. pivot transfer
  D. lift (Hoyer or other brand name)

550. In transfer planning the therapist should, in relationship to her/his own strength, size, and weight,
  A. utilize the best transfer method because her/his own strength, size, and weight have little to do with the correct method
  B. protect her/his own back and body because the correct method of transfer is important but accidents can occur
  C. always have an aide or another therapist nearby to assist in case of an emergency
  D. teach transfer only to family or aides because the risk of getting hurt is too great relative to other people's needs

551. In planning a specific transfer method the therapist uses one method and, in so doing, finds the person slipping from the support given. The therapist should
   A. hold the person up at all costs and complete the transfer
   B. ease the person to the floor and call for help
   C. ease the person to the floor and cushion the fall with his/her own body
   D. hold the person up and call for help

QUESTIONS 552–556: For a person in a wheelchair, accessories are important for safety, comfort, and function. Select the function most appropriate for the accessory.

552. The detachable arms are most necessary for
   A. ease to get up to a desk or table
   B. a depression transfer
   C. easy mobility on the chair
   D. a lift transfer

553. The desk arms are most necessary for
   A. ease to get up to a desk or table
   B. a depression transfer
   C. easy mobility on the chair
   D. a lift transfer

554. The traction foot plate is used
   A. if the person's feet slide off the pedals
   B. if the person has excessive clonus
   C. if the person wishes to make a forward transfer
   D. if the person wishes to readjust herself/himself back up into the chair

555. The detachable leg rest is ordered
   A. if the person's feet slide off the pedals
   B. if the person has excessive clonus
   C. if the person wishes to make a forward transfer
   D. if the person wishes to readjust herself/himself back up into the chair

556. Toe loops may be needed
    A. if the person's feet slide off the pedals
    B. if the person has excessive clonus
    C. if the person wishes to make a forward transfer
    D. if the person wishes to readjust herself/himself back up into the chair

---

QUESTIONS 557–594: Select the **one** most appropriate answer.

557. In planning independence for a person who is in a wheelchair, the therapist should know that the person needs to conquer curbs. Which method should be used in going up a curb?
    A. Approach the curb backward, let the large back wheel tough the curb, lean backward, and propel the large wheels onto the curb; then keep going backward until the casters are over the curb
    B. Approach the curb forward, move the casters to curb, and pull back quickly on the handrails to raise the casters up and over the curb; lean forward, propel the large wheels onto the curb, and go forward until the wheelchair is away from the curb
    C. Approach the curb forward, move the casters to the curb, and pull back quickly on the handrails to raise the casters up and over the curb; lean backward, propel the large wheels onto the curb, and go forward until the wheelchair is away from the curb
    D. Approach the curb backward, let the large back wheels touch the curb, lean forward, and propel the large wheels onto the curb; then lean backward, and propel the large wheels until the casters clear the curb and move away from it.

558. A person who has suffered an injury resulting in quadriplegia and wishes to be a potential candidate for driver training will do better, on the average, if the injury is at the
   A. C3 level and below
   B. C4 level and below
   C. C5 level and below
   D. C6 level and below

559. In planning for a person who has become handicapped and who has homemaking and child care responsibilities after discharge, a therapist should know that these tasks, even with adaptations, will
   A. require no more energy than previously
   B. require an even greater expenditure of energy than before
   C. require that some previous homemaking activities be dropped
   D. require that most previous homemaking activities be dropped

560. In planning for energy conservation for the person in Question 559, the therapist should realize that even with modifications but without proper training the person
   A. may consume an amount of energy in doing daily tasks disproportionate to that required before
   B. may consume the same amount of energy in doing daily tasks as required before
   C. may not consume any more energy in daily tasks than required before
   D. may consume in doing daily tasks two to three times the energy required before

561. In the planning for a handicapped homemaker the therapist should be skilled in demonstrating techniques to that person. The best technique seems to be to
    A. demonstrate the skill to be used in a similar occupational therapy activity
    B. demonstrate the skill as closely as possible to the manner in which it will be used
    C. demonstrate the skill needed and have the person watch
    D. let the person demonstrate the skill needed the best way he or she possibly can

562. In demonstrating a technique to the handicapped homemaker, the therapist should sit or stand beside the person while demonstrating the activity to
    A. avoid left-right confusion
    B. give confidence to the person
    C. give assistance immediately if needed
    D. avoid problems of hearing, seeing, and feeling

563. In planning for "older" Americans the therapist should know that the diagnosis "organic brain syndrome" occurs in older persons. Which description comes closest to indicating the percentages of people with this diagnosis that might be encountered?
    A. 10% of people 65-75 years old and 20% of people 75 years old and older
    B. 15% of people 65-75 years old and 25% of people 75 years old and older
    C. 20% of people 65-75 years old and 25% of people 75 years old and older
    D. 25% of people 65-75 years old and 30% of people 75 years old and older

564. Organic brain syndrome is a psychiatric disorder that reflects brain cell loss or impairment of brain tissue function. In planning to work with this group of people, the therapist should know that basic type(s) that will be encountered is
   A. a mixed group with other diagnoses
   B. a chronic group
   C. an acute group
   D. an acute group and a chronic group

565. In planning to work with a person with a senile psychosis, a therapist should be aware that these symptoms are
   A. irreversible
   B. reversible
   C. precursors of greater impairment
   D. episodic and will diminish

566. In planning a treatment program for a person with diabetes mellitus, the therapist should be aware of insulin shock. If an increased exercise program is planned, the therapist, to avoid insulin shock, should
   A. avoid additional time in occupational therapy and plan for rest
   B. avoid excessive verbal discussions of food in occupational therapy
   C. assist the patient in increasing between-meal intake
   D. assist the patient in avoiding any between-meal intake

567. In planning treatment, perhaps the most important aspect to remember is that the consumer should be involved as much as possible with the plan
   A. as soon after its inception as possible
   B. as soon as the staff approves of the plan
   C. as soon as the therapist designs the plan
   D. as soon as the therapist formulates the plan and has it approved by the physician

568. In planning treatment for a person with severe mood swings, the therapist should be aware of the activities to plan for and those to avoid, given that
   A. the depressive reactions are severe symptoms of depression that are attributed to life experiences and the person has a tenuous grip on reality and the ability to function may be greatly impaired
   B. the depressive reactions are most common in older persons and often are initiated by the loss of a loved one, disappointment, criticism, or threats
   C. the depressive reactions may occur as cyclic episodes of mood swings from elation to depression at any time
   D. the depressive reactions are characterized by guilt feelings, reduced self-regard, anxiety, somatic preoccupations, and delusory ideas

569. In planning treatment for a person with a diagnosis of involutional melancholia or involutional psychotic reaction, the therapist should plan activities that would tend to counteract which of the following situations?
   A. The depressive reactions are severe symptoms of depression that are attributed to life experiences and the person has a tenuous grip on reality and the ability to function may be greatly impaired
   B. The depressive reactions are most common in older persons and often are initiated by the loss of a loved one, disappointment, criticism, or threats
   C. The depressive reactions may occur as cyclic episodes of mood swings from elation to depression at anytime
   D. The depressive reactions are characterized by guilt feelings, reduced self-regard, anxiety, somatic preoccupations, and delusory ideas

570. In planning treatment for a person with a psychotic depressive reaction, the therapist should plan activities of a very solid and simple nature for which of the following situations?
    A. The depressive reactions are severe symptoms of depression that are attributed to life experiences and the person has a tenuous grip on reality and the ability to function may be greatly impaired
    B. The depressive reactions are most common in older persons and often are initiated by the loss of a loved one, disappointment, criticism, or threats
    C. The depressive reactions may occur as cyclic episodes of mood swings from elation to depression at anytime
    D. The depressive reactions are characterized by guilt feelings, reduced self-regard, anxiety, somatic preoccupations, and delusory ideas

571. In planning treatment for a person with a diagnosis of a depressive reaction, the therapist should plan to take into consideration which of the following situations?
    A. The depressive reactions are severe symptoms of depression that are attributed to life experiences and the person has a tenuous grip on reality and the ability to function may be greatly impaired
    B. The depressive reactions are most common in older persons and often are initiated by the loss of a loved one, disappointment, criticism, or threats
    C. The depressive reactions may occur as cyclic episodes of mood swings from elation to depression at anytime
    D. The depressive reactions are characterized by guilt feelings, reduced self-regard, anxiety, somatic preoccupations, and delusory ideas

572. In planning a person's goals in the treatment process, the therapist should know that understanding the client's goals is to be
   A. taken into consideration in the overall goals
   B. the first priority in any treatment setting
   C. taken into consideration in view of the therapist's ability
   D. taken into consideration in view of the department's facilities

573. Treatment planning in occupational therapy is
   A. a rigid technical application of an ameliorative procedure for discrete problems
   B. a process of professional judgment that has identified the right course of action for groups of people with similar dysfunctions
   C. a problem-solving process wherein the therapist selects relevant information and integrates it into an explanation of a person's dysfunction
   D. a rather simplistic process of gathering professional judgments from fellow workers and using past professional successes and applying them to the individual person's dysfunction

574. In occupational therapy, treatment planning decisions regarding which goals should be accomplished first are
   A. too often made by the occupational therapist
   B. too often made by the client
   C. too often made according to the occupational therapy department's policies
   D. too often made according to the center's treatment policies

575. In treatment planning, selection of media is based on the
   A. skill of the person for whom goals are selected
   B. skill of the therapist to track the task
   C. activity analysis and the person's style of learning
   D. person's ability to sense the continuum between the activity and its outcome

576. When a student is involved in treatment planning, which should take precedence?
   A. Write detailed plans so as not to miss any steps
   B. Write sketchy plans and fill in as more details arrive
   C. Do not write plans, as most therapists overlook this part of planning
   D. Write plans that parallel those of the therapist who has responsibility for the person involved

577. A therapist has evaluated a person using a projective test based on a psychoanalytical model and plans to implement treatment on the basis of these results. The therapist would start by planning
   A. to work on behavior modifications
   B. to work on the person's defense mechanisms
   C. a detailed learning-education program
   D. a program on occupational dysfunction

578. In the treatment planning process the most difficult step is
   A. development of the treatment objectives
   B. gathering the necessary data about the person
   C. determining if occupational therapy can be employed
   D. making the assumption that the treatment methods will meet the objectives

579. In planning a ROM exam for certain joints, where should the examiner be positioned in relation to the person tested?
   A. Wherever the best anatomical position can be maintained
   B. Squarely in front of the person
   C. On the side of the person where the joint is being measured
   D. Wherever greatest comfort, correct placement of the instrument, and adequate stability of the joint can be obtained

580. In planning for the development of strength of a specific individual muscle, the most precise method is
   A. using a functional muscle test including the specific muscle
   B. testing the individual muscles
   C. testing groups of muscles and looking for specific motions
   D. observing ordinary activities and movement patterns that use the individual muscle

581. In planning to use a manual muscle test on a person with a lower motor neuron disorder to increase muscle strength, the student should be aware of which limitation of the test?
   A. It is a primary evaluation tool for such persons
   B. Its results test for muscle contractions and range of motion
   C. It measures muscle endurance and coordination
   D. Its validity depends on careful observations and positioning

582. The student in planning to use a manual muscle test must consider gravity as a form of resistance. Which of the following must be considered as a limitation in the test?
   A. Muscle grade is determined whether or not a muscle can move the part against the gravity
   B. Gravity-eliminated positions and movements are parallel to the floor
   C. Gravity-assisted movements are toward the floor and are never used in testing
   D. Movements against gravity are away from the floor and are used in testing

583. In planning treatment for a person with hypotonic muscles, the therapist should know that the ROM test will show
   A. an unusually wide ROM
   B. an average ROM
   C. a limited ROM
   D. no response to a ROM

584. In planning treatment for a person with spasticity, the therapist should know that
    A. a standardized method exists for evaluation of muscle tone
    B. no standardized method exists for evaluation of muscle tone
    C. evaluation of muscle tone falls in an average category
    D. evaluation of muscle tone can largely be ignored

585. In planning treatment for a person with rigidity, the therapist should know that evaluation of the ROM will show that
    A. the agonistic and antagonistic muscle groups contract steadily
    B. the agonistic and antagonistic muscle groups work with a "clasp-knife" phenomenon
    C. the agonistic muscle group works with a jerk immediately followed by the jerk of the antagonistic group
    D. co-contraction of the agonistic and antagonistic muscle groups is weak or absent

586. In planning treatment for a person who will return to his/her former occupation but has symptoms of anosmia the therapist should be aware that
    A. persons with receptive aphasia can be tested with validity
    B. return of a person with a distorted sense of smell to their work site may place him/her in jeopardy
    C. distortion of the sense of smell might not interfere with perception or other factors at the work place
    D. testing of persons with anosmia provides objective criteria on which to plan ahead

587. For a person with rheumatoid arthritis with involvement of the wrist metacarpophalangeal (MP) and interphalangeal (IP) joints, a volar resting splint is indicated
   A. to improve hand function and grip strength when the hand function is limited by wrist pain
   B. to protect the MP joints from ulnar deviation and the forces of volar subluxation
   C. when there is acute synovitis of the wrist, fingers, and thumb
   D. when both the wrist and MP joints are involved

588. For a person with rheumatoid arthritis with involvement of the wrist MP and IP joints, a wrist stabilization splint is indicated
   A. to improve hand function and grip strength when the hand function is limited by wrist pain
   B. to protect the MP joints from ulnar deviation and the forces of volar subluxation
   C. when there is acute synovitis of the wrist, fingers, and thumb
   D. when both the wrist and MP joints are involved

589. For a person with rheumatoid arthritis with involvement of the wrist MP and IP joints, a protective MP splint is indicated
   A. to improve hand function and grip strength when the hand function is limited by wrist pain
   B. to protect the MP joints from ulnar deviation and the forces of volar subluxation
   C. when there is acute synovitis of the wrist, fingers, and thumb
   D. when both the wrist and MP joints are involved

590. In planning treatment for a person with rheumatoid arthritis who has a swan-neck deformity at the distal interphalangeal (DIP) joint, which of the following would the therapist identify as the cause of the deformity and take the necessary precautions in working with that person?
    A. The deformity is a result of rupture of the flexor digitorum sublimis (FDS) tendon
    B. The deformity is a result of rupture or lengthening of the central slip of the extensor digitorum communis (EDC) tendon
    C. The deformity is a result of rupture of the lateral slip of the EDC tendons
    D. The deformity is the result of a module or thickening of the FDS tendon at the flex or tunnel

591. In planning treatment for a person with rheumatoid arthritis who has a swan-neck deformity at the proximal interphalangeal (PIP) joint, which of the following would the therapist identify as the cause of the deformity and take the necessary precautions in working with that person?
    A. The deformity is a result of rupture of the FDS tendon
    B. The deformity is a result of rupture or lengthening of the central slip of the EDC tendon
    C. The deformity is a result of rupture of the lateral slip of the EDC tendons
    D. The deformity is the result of a module or thickening of the FDS tendon at the flex or tunnel

592. In planning treatment for a person with rheumatoid arthritis who has a boutonniere deformity at the PIP joint, which of the following would the therapist identify as the cause of the deformity and take the necessary precautions in working with that person?
    A. The deformity is a result of rupture of the FDS tendon
    B. The deformity is a result of rupture or lengthening of the central slip of the EDC tendon
    C. The deformity is a result of rupture of the lateral slip of the EDC tendons
    D. The deformity is the result of a module or thickening of the FDS tendon at the flex or tunnel

593. In planning a ROM program for a person who has had a severe head injury, the therapist must know that
   A. most adults have muscle weakness
   B. a person may start with flaccid muscles and rapidly develop severe spasticity
   C. most adults have normal muscle strength
   D. a person may usually have severe extensor patterning of the upper extremities and flexor patterning of the lower extremities

594. Abnormal postural reflexes such as ATNR, STNR, and TCR are common problems usually found in people suffering from head injuries. In planning a ROM program the therapist must know that
   A. unless prevented or controlled, these abnormal reflexes will eventually come back to normal after the severity of the injury wears off
   B. unless prevented or controlled, these abnormal reflexes may prevent the person from making even basic physical and functional gains
   C. the brain-injured person has the same clinical picture as the person with a CVA and the same ROM pattern will return in the same general time period
   D. even though one or all four extremities may be involved a ROM program should plan on the progress of extremities from proximal to distal

QUESTIONS 595–599: Kathleen L. Reed details many descriptive models for occupational therapists' use in working with people who have psychiatric dysfunction. The models from the late 1950s into the 1970s are based upon certain frames of reference.

595. A therapist planning to use the "object relations" modal should know that this model is
   A. based primarily on Lewin's concept of life space but enlarged to include the forces of the community, specifically of time, space, resources, and relationships
   B. based on concepts of a therapeutic community or milieu therapy and group dynamics and, further, on the premise that many mental health problems are the result of failure to learn to function in the community
   C. based on Freudian psychoanalysis, which is in turn based on the mechanistic model
   D. not based on any specific school of thought, but the concepts and assumptions of Freudian psychoanalysis are clearly evident

596. A therapist planning to use the "activity therapy" model should know that this model is
   A. based primarily on Lewin's concept of life space but enlarged to include the forces of the community, specifically of time, space, resources, and relationships
   B. based on concepts of a therapeutic community or milieu therapy and group dynamics and, further, on the premise that many mental health problems are the result of failure to learn to function in the community
   C. based on Freudian psychoanalysis, which is in turn based on the mechanistic model
   D. not based on any specific school of thought, but the concepts and assumptions of Freudian psychoanalysis are clearly evident

597. A therapist planning to use the "communication process" model should know that this model was
   A. based primarily on Lewin's concept of life space but enlarged to include the forces of the community, specifically of time, space, resources, and relationships
   B. based on concepts of a therapeutic community or milieu therapy and group dynamics and, further, on the premise that many mental health problems are the result of failure to learn to function in the community
   C. based on Freudian psychoanalysis, which is in turn based on the mechanistic model
   D. not based on any specific school of thought, but the concepts and assumptions of Freudian psychoanalysis are clearly evident

598. In planning for a child with a chronic disability, the therapist must be aware that the model of human occupation provides a useful framework for planning and subsequent treatment. It compels the therapist to view the child as
   A. an open system
   B. a closed system
   C. a long-term (chronic) system
   D. a dependent system

599. In planning a program using the model of human occupation, the therapist must examine which of the following perspectives in order to prevent becoming preoccupied with the pathology of the child?
   A. the parents' or family's view of chronicity
   B. the child's view of his or her own chronicity
   C. his or her own view of chronicity
   D. the team's overall view of chronicity

Explanatory Answers

500. (B) There seems to be enough evidence to conclude that activities are characteristic of a state of humanness and that the body and mind are enhanced in using activities. Therefore it is assumed that different kinds of activities have a role to play in the development of a physically sound and well-integrated personality. (REF. 10, p. 13)

501. (C) In addition to the above, there is evidence that utilization of activities seems to provide a person with the means of attaining a sense of mastery and well-being. (REF. 10, p. 13)

502. (C) Activities are socioculturally regulated by a system of values and beliefs and thus are defined by (and in turn define) acceptable norms of behavior. (REF. 10, p. 13)

503. (A) The permissible range of activity-related behaviors varies from society to society as well as with respect to age, sex, caste, class, and occupation. (REF. 10, p. 14)

504. (A) The permissible range of activity-related behaviors varies from society to society as well as with respect to age, sex, caste, class, and occupation. (REF. 10, p. 14)

505. (A) We are currently in the midst of a conscious rebellion against a series of prescribed activities that were seen as a norm. Sex-allocated roles are being challenged and today many young people from similar backgrounds do not seem to be greatly concerned about doing the same thing. (REF. 10, p. 15)

506. (C) One fundamental assumption about the nature of humankind is that individuals can change and indeed desire change. (REF. 10, p. 15)

507. (B) It is evident that a number of specific activities fit quite appropriately into one or more categories; for example, eating could be classified as a self-care activity, a social activity, or a work-related activity, as in the preparation of food. (REF. 10, p. 20)

508. (D) The notion of activities in a field of action provides for structuring activities so that they simulate, as nearly as possible, conditions in the real world. (REF. 10, p. 21)

509. (C) Activities in a field of action follow rules that govern the conduct of specific activities from both implicit and explicit means that occur either before or during an activity. (REF. 10, p. 21)

510. (A) To achieve a sense of accomplishment or competence, a task requires that it have some beginning and some end. (REF. 10, p. 36)

511. (A) An activity that is approved as appropriate by age group and sex must have some meaningful structure to it if it requires skill that is a little beyond that possessed by the person doing it. (REF. 10, p. 36)

512. (B) The "teacher"-therapist must be a day-to-day working model with whom to interact, not a model to imitate, with interaction, liking, and respect most likely following. (REF. 10, p. 36)

513. (D) Activities are therapeutic when they enable change to take place in a direction from dysfunction to function. (REF. 10, p. 38)

514. (A) Activities will enable change to take place in an individual if the activity has meaning and relevance to the individual who is to change. (REF. 10, p. 38)

515. (C) Activities will enable change to take place if they are based upon systematically organized and administered principles derived from a methodical treatment approach based on a theoretical rationale or empirical evidence. (REF. 10, p. 38)

516. (B) It is possible to probe in greater depth the meaning of activities and their worth to a person by using an exploratory tool such as an activity inventory, which will produce a chronological listing of specific activities that have helped form a pattern of the individual's everyday life. (REF. 10, p. 39)

517. (C) Principles of planning include the establishment of goals that meet client's needs but also can be realistically carried out within the constraints of the therapeutic situation. (REF. 10, p. 69)

518. (B) There may be times when both long-range overall goals and short-term goals merge. (REF. 10, p. 69)

519. (A) One of the principles in planning is to use the simplest and least amount of equipment possible to effect maximal function. (REF. 10, p. 69)

520. (C) Another principle of planning is to schedule activities with sufficient frequency of repetition and duration to ensure integration of learning. (REF. 10, p. 70)

521. (B) Yet another principle of planning is to schedule specific periods of evaluation of progress. (REF. 10, p. 70)

522. (A) More personal energy is needed and spent by older persons in the care and maintenance of the body. Therefore, more independence must be relinquished as one becomes increasingly dependent upon others to perform services that previously had been done by the individual. (REF. 19, p. 31)

523. (A) Physical changes occur in older persons. More energy is used just to care and maintain the body. Because of these concerns whole new patterns of life need to be initiated. (REF. 19, p. 31)

524. (C) As an older person's social world begins to diminish, separation from the community and loneliness often become an established consequence. (REF. 19, p. 31)

525. (B) Geriatric specialists should be knowledgeable about the latest legislative programs offered to older persons so that they can inform these people of the services available to them and have a more thorough understanding of current funding sources. (REF. 19, p. 40)

526. (A) Since most older people experience at least two chronic

527. (A) diseases simultaneously, it is essential that in planning treatment the therapist acquire firm knowledge of the diseases most prevalent among the elderly. (REF. 19, p. 59)

528. (C) A reality orientation program is based upon the assumption that repetition of basic information such as name, day, place, date, and other events can reinforce learning and ameliorate disorientation and confusion. (REF. 19, p. 62)

529. (B) Attitude therapy is helpful in reinforcing desirable behavior and eliminating undesirable behavior. It often is used in conjunction with reality orientation programs. (REF. 19, p. 63)

530. (D) Remotivation is a technique usually begun after successful completion of a reality orientation program. Remotivation is used to encourage moderately confused older people to become more interested in their surroundings and environment by focusing attention on simple objective topics not seemingly related to that person's emotional problems. (REF. 19, p. 64)

531. (C) A formal reality orientation program usually consists of four or five class members and an instructor. They meet at the same time at least five days per week and continue until the class graduates. (REF. 19, p. 61)

532. (A) Attitude therapy involves a consistent rehabilitation team approach consisting of five major attitudes, one of which is team decided for one individual. Everyone coming into contact with this client utilizes the designated attitude, and it persists until a change occurs. (REF. 19, p. 6)

533. (B) Remotivation is a technique that usually follows the successful completion of a reality orientation program. A series generally continues for 12 weeks, with one 30- to 60-minute session per week. The group consists of 5 to 12 people and makes use of a 5-point outline in a semiformal manner. (REF. 19, p. 6)

534. (A) Since therapeutic crafts often are misunderstood by the people utilizing them and other professionals, it is a paramount obligation of the therapist to seize every opportunity to explain arts and crafts and how a specific craft is to be used to eliminate a person's dysfunction. (REF. 19, p. 95)

535. (A) The modern concept of death is very different from ancient beliefs. Technology and other factors are responsible for new attitudes toward death. Today our society tends to transpose death from an immediate and perpetual menace to one of remote possibility. (REF. 19, p. 101)

536. (B) Social scientists believe that the fear of death is universal and that (perhaps because of death's certainty) Americans seem to cope by using mechanisms such as avoidance, denial, and repudiation. (REF. 19, p. 103)

537. (B) Kubler-Ross believes there are six stages of death and dying, beginning with denial and, all things being equal, ending with acceptance. (REF. 19, p. 103)

538. (A) Jeffers and Verwoerdt affirm that seven factors are critical in determining the type of coping techniques that an individual can use when facing death, starting with chronological age and distance from death and ending with the individual's psychological maturity and integrity. (REF. 19, p. 103)

539. (C) Weisman (in *On Dying and Denying: A Psychiatric Study of Terminality*) postulates that death from old age consists of six phases, starting with repudiation of growing older and ending with cessation of life. (REF. 19, p. 103)

540. (B) A professional team agreed that in the area of death and dying most health care professionals impose emotional isolation upon dying persons, treat them in a routine manner, and handle them as if they were irresponsible children who cannot cope with the situation on an adult level. (REF. 19, p. 104)

541. (A) To decrease a behavior without offering a constructive alternative behavior leaves the person to his/her own devices. New behavior may not be any more socially acceptable than original behavior, so one should attempt to increase acceptable behavior when decreasing unacceptable behavior. (REF. 10, p. 52)

542. (B) The psychiatric treatment plan should be developed in collaboration with the client so that some degree of mutual understanding about the occupational therapy process can be arrived at by both the therapist and the person for whom the plan was designed. (REF. 15, p. 308)

543. (C) Treatment plans represent a synthesis of the therapist's knowledge of the potential of activities and their relationships as facilitators of growth and performance. (REF. 15, p. 309)

544. (B) The therapist should maintain the attitude that the person for whom the goals are formulated has the right to determine her/his own life goals. (REF. 18, p. 152)

545. (C) No matter what the future holds or what the prognosis of a given person is, everyone assigned to occupational therapy deserves the best that can be offered. (REF. 18, p. 153)

546. (A) A sliding transfer is designed for a person who is unable to bear weight on the lower extremities or has weak upper extremities. (REF. 16, p. 459)

547. (D) A lift (Hoyer or otherwise) is planned for a person who cannot move his/her own body. (REF. 16, p. 459)

548. (B) A depression transfer is appropriate for a person who is unable to bear weight on the lower extremities but has strong enough upper extremities to lift his/her weight off a surface. (REF. 16, p. 459)

549. (C) A pivot transfer is used if weight bearing on the lower extremities is either possible or permitted. (REF. 16, p. 459)

550. (B) When involved in any transfer of another person, the therapist must protect his/her own back and body. (REF. 16, p. 459)

551. (C) Should a therapist overestimate his/her own strength or underestimate the weight of a person, and should that person start to slip during the transfer, the therapist should ease that person to the floor and use his/her own body to cushion the fall. (REF. 16, p. 459)

552. (B) Detachable arms are necessary for depression or sliding transfers. (REF. 16, p. 303)

553. (A) Desk arms enable a person's chair to move close to a table or desk. (REF. 16, p. 303)

554. (A) Traction foot plates are ordered if a person's feet have a tendency to slip off the pedals. (REF. 16, p. 304)

555. (C) A detachable leg rest is required if a forward transfer is necessary into a tub or where a slide transfer is not possible. (REF. 16, p. 303)

556. (B) The toe loop may be needed when a person has excessive clonus and cannot keep her/his feet on the pedals. (REF. 16, p. 304)

557. (B) To go up a curb on a wheelchair, approach the curb forward. As the casters near the curb, pull back quickly on the handrails to raise the front of the chair onto the curb, lean forward, and propel the back wheels onto the curb. (REF. 16, p. 462)

558. (D) A person with a diagnosis of quadriplegia in whom the injury occurred at the C6 level of below is considered a potential candidate for driver training. (REF. 16, p. 477)

559. (B) Homemaking and child care activities are energy-consuming for anyone. But a disabled person who must use adapted methods will find that an even greater expenditure of energy is needed. (REF. 16, p. 480)

560. (A) Unless a handicapped homemaker is trained in the modification of daily tasks, that person may use a disproportionate amount of energy. (REF. 16, p. 480)

561. (B) The therapist should be skilled in demonstrating a technique in a way that is as close as possible to the manner in which the disabled person will be expected to do it. (REF. 16, p. 481)

562. (A) While instructing a person about an activity, the therapist should sit or stand beside the person to eliminate right-left confusion. (REF. 16, p. 481)

563. (B) About 15% of people 65 to 75 years of age and 25% of people over 75 years of age have been diagnosed as having organic brain syndrome. (REF. 19, p. 45)

564. (D) Organic brain syndrome is a psychiatric disorder that can be classified as one of two basic types: (1) acute or reversible and (2) chronic or irreversible. (REF. 19, p. 46)

565. (C) Senile psychosis is a progressive decline in mental functioning associated with errors in judgment, decline in self-care habits, loosening of inhibitions, impairment of abstract thought, and many other behaviors. These symptoms are precursors of greater impairment. (REF. 19, p. 47)

566. (C) To avoid insulin shock the diabetic must account for an increase in exercise or routing by a corresponding increase in between-meal intake. (REF. 19, p. 58)

567. (A) Perhaps the most important aspect to remember about treatment planning is that the consumer should be involved as much as possible from its inception. (REF. 19, p. 61)

568. (C) For a person with severe mood swings, the therapist should plan activities that can be quickly adjusted to meet the mood swings from elation to depression. (REF. 19, p. 42)

569. (D) For a person with an involutional melancholia, the therapist should be aware that guilt feelings, reduced self-respect, anxiety, somatic preoccupation, agitation, and delusory ideas are associated with this person's illness, and should make plans accordingly. (REF. 19, p. 42)

570. (A) For a person with a psychotic depressive reaction, the therapist should plan activities that take into consideration the fact that the severe symptoms of this person can be attributed to a definable life experience. In such a state the person has only a tenuous grip on reality, and the ability to function may be greatly impaired. Thus, only a solid approach with simple activities should be attempted. (REF. 19, p. 42)

571. (B) For a person with a depressive reaction (depressive neurosis), the therapist should know that this diagnosis is the most common neurosis of older persons. It is often initiated by the loss of a loved one, disappointment in life goals, criticism, or threats, and the therapist should plan a program to avoid involvement in these areas if that is part of the overall plan. (REF. 19, p. 42)

572. (B) Understanding the client's goals is the first priority in any therapeutic setting. Therapists should be cognizant of the client's grasp of reality. (REF. 19, p. 162)

573. (C) Treatment planning is a problem-solving process in which the therapist selects relevant information about a person's unique function or dysfunction and also uses a process of professional judgment that identifies the right course of action. (REF. 20, p. 136)

574. (A) Program planning goals are too often made by the therapist or the treatment team without consulting the client for whom the goals are set. The client may have unrealistic goals, and obtainable goals must be identified and worked toward. (REF. 18, p. 85)

575. (C) Selection of media is based on styles of learning, an activity analysis, the goals desired, media available, and the interest of the person involved. (REF. 18, p. 85)

576. (A) Students need to write detailed plans so that they do not miss any steps and so that the supervising therapist can check their progress and see how well they apply a problem-solving approach. (REF. 18, p. 85)

Planning / 161

577. (B) The philosophy and theory of a therapist and an institution need to be consistent. If a therapist evaluates a person using a projective test based upon a psychoanalytical model and wishes to plan treatment, it would most likely involve working on defense mechanisms and inner conflicts, which are parts of this model. Other models of treatment would not be understood or, perhaps, accepted by the institution or peers. (REF. 18, p. 87)

578. (D) When treatment objectives have been planned, the most difficult step in the process is knowing that the treatment methods will help the client achieve the objectives. (REF. 21, p. 23)

579. (D) The examiner in a ROM exam should position himself/herself and the subject for greatest comfort, correct placement of the instrument, and adequate stability of the joint being measured. (REF. 21, p. 37)

580. (B) the most precise method of developing the strength of an individual muscle is evaluation of that individual muscle, not grouping it with others or observing its function and proceeding to strengthening it. (REF. 21, p. 53)

581. (C) A manual muscle test is a means of measuring maximal contractions of muscles, to determine power, and is a primary evaluation tool for clients with lower motor neuron disorders. Its limitations are that it cannot measure muscle endurance, muscle coordination, or smooth rhythmic interaction of muscle functions. (REF. 21, p. 55)

582. (C) Gravity is a form of resistance to muscle power. A gravity-assisted movement is toward the floor and should not be used in the testing procedure. (REF. 21, p. 55)

583. (A) Hypotonic muscles feel soft and flabby and offer less resistance to passive movement than normal muscles. Because of this laxity the ROM may be unusually wide. (REF. 21, p. 87)

584. (B) Spasticity is usually evaluated by estimating the degree of resistance to passive movement of a given muscle group or pattern of movement. There is no standardized method of evaluating muscle tone with absolute objectivity. (REF. 21, p. 87)

585. (A) Rigidity is an increase in tone of agonistic and antagonistic muscles simultaneously; both groups contract steadily, resulting in an increased resistance to passive movement in any direction throughout the ROM. (REF. 21, p. 89)

586. (B) The loss of smell is known as anosmia. The sense of smell is critical to safety, and when it is distorted it may interfere with perception. Its testing results in subjective data, and persons with receptive aphasia cannot be validly tested. (REF. 21, p. 103)

587. (C) A volar resting splint is indicated when there is acute synovitis of the wrist, fingers, and thumb. Its purpose is to rest the joints and thus decrease inflammation. (REF. 21, p. 296)

588. (A) A wrist stabilization splint is indicated to immobilize the wrist but allow motion of the MP joints. It is used when hand function is limited by wrist pain, and improves hand function and grip strength. (REF. 21, p. 296)

589. (B) The protective MP splint is indicated to maintain the MP joints in normal alignment and protect the joints from ulnar deviation and the forces of volar subluxation. (REF. 21, p. 296)

590. (C) The swan-neck deformity at the DIP joint is a result of rupture of the lateral slip of the EDC tendons. (REF. 21, p. 301)

591. (A) A swan-neck deformity with involvement at the PIP joint is caused by rupture of the FDS tendon. (REF. 21, p. 301)

592. (B) The boutonniere deformity is caused by a rupture or lengthening of the central slip of the EDC tendon. (REF. 20, p. 301)

593. (B) A person with a severe head injury may have one or all extremities involved. It is extremely important in the early stages to control loss of ROM. A person may start out with flaccid muscles and quickly develop severe spasticity and deformities. A person may usually have severe flex or patterning of the lower extremities. (REF. 21, p. 438)

594. (B) Abnormal postural reflexes are a common problem found in people suffering from head injuries. These abnormal reflexes and reactions affect ROM. Unless prevented or controlled, they may prevent the person from making even basic physical and functional gains. The clinical pictures of CVA and brain injury are not the same, and return of controlled movement usually is from proximal to distal, although at times it can occur distal to proximal. (REF. 21, p. 438)

595. (C) The Ozimos (Dr. H. and Fran) developed the "object relations" model based on Freudian psychoanalysis, which in turn is based on the mechanistic model. (REF. 22, p. 384)

596. (B) Dr. Ann C. Mosey developed the "activity therapy" model based on the concept of a therapeutic community or milieu therapy and group dynamics. (REF. 22, p. 421)

597. (D) Although the Fidlers (Dr. Jay and Gail) stated that the "communication process" model was not based on any specific school of thought, the concepts and assumptions of Freudian psychoanalysis are clearly evident in their work. (REF. 22, p. 389)

598. (A) The model of human occupation provides a useful framework for therapists and compels them to see chronic disabilities in children as an open system and as a focus away from specific pathology. (REF. 20, p. 329)

599. (C) It is important, at the onset of planning a program under the model of human occupation, for a therapist to examine his/her own perspective of people with chronic disabilities. All clinicians are in danger of becoming preoccupied with pathology, and the child, being vulnerable, could absorb this pathology-centered attitude as his or her own. (REF. 20, p. 329)

8 Implementation

QUESTIONS 600 and 601: Select the **one** most appropriate answer.

600. In children with dysfunctions from birth, the younger the child the greater the potential for treatment because
    A. the central nervous system is still developing and primitive patterns are not strongly developed
    B. no injury to the central nervous system has occurred, and therefore it is still intact
    C. families with youngsters are more eager and willing to assist in the overall treatment plan, especially after-care
    D. psychological components of both the young child and the family have not been damaged by long-term chronicity and thus are easier to work with

601. Treatment plans designed for motor function in a child with severe damage of long standing may have the therapist
    A. exercise for gross motor patterns
    B. utilize primitive reflexes for locomotion
    C. inhibit reflexes so higher functions are promoted first
    D. evaluate upper extremities for utilization of an electric wheelchair

QUESTIONS 602–605: In implementing treatment for people with disturbances of coordination, the therapist notices the conditions listed (lettered). Match the condition with its description.

- **A.** Tremor
- **B.** Dysdiadochokinesia
- **C.** Decomposition of movement
- **D.** Dysmetria

602. There is an impaired ability to accomplish repeated alternating movements rapidly and smoothly such as alternate supination-pronation of the forearm.
603. There is an extreme amount of movement during a planned movement and diminished or absent movement during rest.
604. There is an ability to control muscle length, which results in overshooting, such as trying to touch the face and hitting the face instead.
605. Each joint in a person's movement pattern functions independently so that the movement is broken up into parts rather than being smooth and coordinated.

Implementation / 167

QUESTIONS 606–609: In implementing treatment for persons with basal ganglia lesions or disease the therapist notices the conditions listed (lettered). Match the condition with its description.

A. Athetosis
B. Chorea
C. Dystonia
D. Tremor

606. The person demonstrates rapid, jerky, irregular movements, involving primarily the face and distal extremities.
607. When the person is at rest, rapid movements begin; but when the person works at an activity, the excessive movements disappear.
608. Movement about the neck, face, and extremities is characterized as slow, writhing, twisting, and wormlike.
609. A person demonstrates a distorted posture of the trunk and extremities.

QUESTIONS 610–625: Select the **one** most appropriate answer.

610. The therapist begins treatment of a new person who, after a few minutes, starts a violent, forceful, flinging movement of the extremities on the left side of the body, particularly involving the proximal musculature. The therapist reports that the person has
A. right CVA
B. epilepsy
C. hemiballismus
D. hemiparesis

611. A student is working with a person who has rheumatoid arthritis. The student asks the person to flex and extend the fingers. The person attempts to do this, but the fingers droop. The student reports to the supervisor that the person has
    A. tendon ruptures at the metacarpophalangeal joints
    B. a volar subluxation of the hand
    C. an interphalangeal hyperextension
    D. a Landsmeer's ligament, boutonniere deformity

612. A student plans a treatment program for a person with rheumatoid arthritis to maintain or increase mobility of joints and strength in the hands. The therapist approves the plan. The student starts the plan, but the person complains of pain. The therapist suggests that the student
    A. disregard the pain because the increase in mobility and development of strength are more important at this time
    B. continue with the plan to the limit of pain for each joint, but work with each joint at a different time
    C. continue with the plan to the limit of pain for each joint at one period, with the remainder of the day for rest
    D. disregard the pain because the person is well known in the occupational therapy section as a chronic complainer

613. In the preceding situation the therapist makes a second suggestion to the student so that the pain can be reduced and the student can be more relaxed. The therapist suggests that the student
    A. talk to the person and explain the reason for the treatment and that pain is a natural process
    B. let the person come to occupational therapy and rest for the first few minutes before treatment starts
    C. find a simple activity that the person likes, and let him/her do it carefully while monitoring the activity
    D. warm the hand by some method for a period of time before starting treatment

614. If a person in treatment who has rheumatoid arthritis does not have a full active ROM in the hand, a passive ROM to just beyond the point of pain may be necessary. Using a paraffin bath would reduce the pain. The therapist knows the pain should not persist for how many hours after treatment without reducing the next treatment or having the joints rest?
   A. 0-1 hour
   B. 1-2 hours
   C. 2-3 hours
   D. 3-4 hours

615. A student is assigned to and is working with a person who has had a fairly recent traumatic spinal cord injury. The person talks of walking out of the center in the next couple of months. The student knows that as soon as the spinal shock subsides, return of motor functions begins and continues for approximately
   A. 2-4 months, so the person is about right
   B. 4-8 months, so the person is not too far off
   C. 8-10 months, so the person has some time to recover
   D. 11-12 months, so the person has a much longer time to wait

616. In working with the person who has sustained a severe burn, the occupational therapist becomes involved very early in the treatment process by
   A. increasing independence in daily life tasks
   B. increasing endurance
   C. assisting the person in dealing with psychological reactions to pain
   D. positioning to prevent deformity by splinting

617. A student new at a field work experience placement is assigned to a person who has had a myocardial infarction. The student asks if the department has telemetry and electrocardiogram monitoring. The therapist states that
   A. televisions are not permitted in the occupational therapy service area
   B. telemetry and electrocardiogram monitoring are new procedures unavailable at this center
   C. telemetry and electrocardiogram monitoring are not part of occupational therapy work responsibility
   D. telemetry and electrocardiogram monitoring are too new to bother with because they have not been proven to work

618. In planning a cardiac rehabilitation program for a person the therapist should encourage the view that successful recovery from the myocardial infarction leads to a relatively normal and productive life. To assist in accomplishing this goal the therapist will need to educate the
   A. occupational therapy student
   B. treatment team
   C. patient
   D. patient and the family

619. In planning treatment for a person who needs to strengthen shoulder flexors the student notes that the person previously indicated a strong interest in and desire for exercise. With this idea in mind the student suggests that simply sanding blocks of wood would be a good treatment plan. The therapist supervisor states that
   A. this plan is lacking in that any activity selected should have a reasonable end product
   B. this is a good exercise for shoulder strengthening, and when the wood is sanded the person can put it together and make something out of it
   C. this is a good plan as long as the person is concerned about exercise and informed that this activity is only for exercise
   D. this plan is lacking because pure exercise is what the physical therapist does, whereas occupational therapists do activities

620. After 2 weeks of treatment the therapist asks the student to do a motor analysis of an activity. The student quickly asks if the motor analysis should be made from a biomechanical or a neurodevelopmental point of view. The therapist quickly responds that
   A. there is only one way to do it
   B. the biomechanical point of view is the best, so do that one
   C. the neurodevelopmental point of view is the best, so do that one
   D. either one is a good approach, so give me your reasons as to why you want to do one or the other

621. The student wishes to do a motor analysis of a person in treatment to make an objective evaluation of the person's progress. In planning a biomechanical analysis the student should
   A. observe from which side an object is picked up
   B. position the object to be used in exact places
   C. observe whether the object's use demands stability and/or mobility responses and out of which joints
   D. place a number of objects in front of the person to see which one is chosen

622. In the preceding situation the student starts the biomechanical analysis using a clinical approach: observation, palpation, and deduction based on anatomical and kinesiological data. The therapist indicates that in a few weeks the department will have equipment delivered to it so that the student can do more exact measurements. The equipment will be
   A. EMG equipment
   B. EEG equipment
   C. ECG equipment
   D. ECT equipment

623. A student who wishes to do a neurodevelopmental analysis of an activity during treatment will
   A. observe if the person's primitive reflexes are being reinforced
   B. observe if the person is enjoying and receiving benefit from the activity
   C. ask the person what his/her interests and activities are
   D. ask the person to select an activity of his/her own choice

624. In analyzing an activity to determine if it is therapeutically appropriate, a student often watches to see if it is related to the developmental levels and if the potential of the activity provides meaningful opportunities for the individual to develop competence and balance within his or her role in society. This type of analysis is
   A. neurodevelopmental
   B. psychiatric
   C. sensory integrative
   D. occupational behavior

625. In analyzing an activity to determine if it is therapeutically appropriate, a student often watches to see what if any sensory, perceptual, or physical aspects of activity are present. This type of an analysis is
   A. neurodevelopmental
   B. psychiatric
   C. sensory integrative
   D. occupational behavior

QUESTIONS 626–629: In using an activity on a flat surface (such as using finger paint, sanding, or using an exercise skate), the therapist asks the student to change the work surface to accomplish certain functions. Match the change the student needs to make on the work surface with the function to be accomplished.

A. Raise the work surface to axilla height
B. Incline the work surface up
C. Incline the work surface down
D. Lower the work surface to elbow height

626. To accomplish increased resistance to shoulder extension and elbow flexion.
627. To accomplish increased resistance to shoulder flexion and elbow extension.
628. To accomplish flexion and extension of the elbow on a gravity-eliminated plane.
629. To accomplish supination-pronation movements and eliminate shoulder rotation by allowing the upper arm to remain adducted.

QUESTIONS 630–636: Select the one most appropriate answer.

630. In the treatment of people who have chronic illness wherein the goal is independence in self-care, workers hypothesize an order of regaining independence. Comparison of this order with child development and anthropological observations seems to reveal
    A. a psychosocial consistency
    B. an ontogenetic consistency
    C. a phylogenetic consistency
    D. an egocentric consistency

631. In the above-described studies of regaining independence in people with chronic illness, which (as a general rule) sequence would be followed (excluding some diagnostic groups that might require modification or change of the order of sequence)?
   A. Feeding, continence, transferring, going to the toilet, dressing, and bathing
   B. Feeding, dressing, bathing, continence, transferring, and going to the toilet
   C. Feeding, transferring, continence, going to the toilet, bathing, and dressing
   D. Feeding, bathing, dressing, transferring, continence, and going to the toilet

632. In the treatment planning for self-care activities the principle of compensation for limited range of joint motion is to
   A. provide stability
   B. change body mechanics or techniques
   C. increase a person's reach
   D. provide substitution for stabilizing

633. In the treatment planning for self-care activities the principle of compensation for incoordination is to
   A. provide stability
   B. change body mechanics or techniques
   C. increase a person's reach
   D. provide substitution for stabilizing

634. In the treatment planning for self-care activities the principle of compensation for decreased strength is to
   A. provide stability
   B. change body mechanics or techniques
   C. increase a person's reach
   D. provide substitution for stabilizing

635. In the treatment planning for self-care activities the principle of compensation for loss of use on one side of the upper extremities is to
   A. provide stability
   B. change body mechanics or techniques
   C. increase a person's reach
   D. provide substitution for stabilizing

636. In treatment planning that invades the home, the therapist should have some basic facts relative to doorways and ramps. For wheelchairs, which measurements are correct for an ideal architectural design for a doorway width (inches), ramp width (inches), and incline (degrees)?
   A. Doorway, 36; ramp, 30 to 40; incline, 1 to 12
   B. Doorway, 34; ramp, 24 to 36; incline, 1 to 6
   C. Doorway, 36; ramp, 24 to 36; incline, 1 to 18
   D. Doorway, 34; ramp, 30 to 40; incline, 1 to 14

QUESTIONS 637–639: Therapeutic approaches to be used with one person or another are organized tasks or activities used in a series of steps based on a system of logic. These approaches are generally understood and easily implemented. Often the disadvantages or major drawbacks of a therapeutic approach are a little harder to understand. Below are some approaches and their disadvantages. Match the correct disadvantage with the correct approach.

   A. The sequence may not be an advantage for a person's handicap
   B. The activity is not useful unless it meets the client's needs
   C. The sequence may increase problems rather than reduce them
   D. Performance does not always occur normally but as an integrated continuous flow of behavioral performance

637. In normal developmental sequencing, tasks are selected according to the normal progression of skills acquired in the average child or adult.

638. In normal activity sequencing, many activities have a logical sequence of steps that facilitate task performance. The steps are not always necessarily invariant, but a sequence may require less total time or a repetition of steps.

639. In a task analysis of a therapeutic approach, each step in a sequence is examined so the therapist can determine which steps a person can or cannot perform.

QUESTIONS 640–699: Select the **one** most appropriate answer.

---

640. Which most closely describes the psychiatric occupational therapy treatment process of intervening directly in the illness of the person?
   A. Dealing with the person's strengths and promotion of optimum abilities
   B. Dealing with the person's strengths and healthy parts
   C. Effecting changes in the pathology
   D. Effecting changes in personality by support and encouragement

641. Another of the psychiatric occupational therapy treatment processes is that of the maintenance of function. Which of the following refers to this process?
   A. Dealing with the person's strengths and promotion of optimum abilities
   B. Dealing with the person's strengths and healthy parts
   C. Effecting changes in the pathology
   D. Effecting changes in personality by support and encouragement

642. A third treatment process is a developmental and occupational frame of reference or a rehabilitation-prevention process. Which of the following refers to this process?
   A. Dealing with the person's strengths and promotion of optimum abilities
   B. Dealing with the person's strengths and healthy parts
   C. Effecting changes in the pathology
   D. Effecting changes in personality by support and encouragement

643. After evaluation and planning have occurred the implementation process starts. It is broken into parts. Which set comprises the parts of the implementation phase?
    A. Orientation, implementation, and termination
    B. Evaluation, implementation, reevaluation, and termination
    C. Evaluation, objective setting, planning, implementation, and termination
    D. Orientation, development, and termination

644. The therapeutic program requires that after implementation begins, the objectives be translated into specific activities. These activities must be relevant to the
    A. objectives and have meaning for the client
    B. physician and team members
    C. hospital's overall plan and objectives
    D. objectives of the occupational therapy service area

645. In a schematic representation of the levels on which activities for people with psychosocial dysfunctions may be experienced, the first of six levels is body awareness experiences where movement and sensory input activities are of value. Which of the following would further guide the selection of activities for this experience level?
    A. Activities may use but are not dependent upon verbal activity, end products, and process
    B. Activities are individual, and process is important, automatic, and noncortical
    C. Activities are primarily nonverbal, and end products are process-oriented and individual
    D. Activities are group-oriented, verbal and nonverbal, and process- and product-oriented

646. In the same schematic representation the second level is body effectiveness experience. Which of the following would further guide the selection of activities for this experience level?
   A. Activities may use but are not dependent upon verbal activity, end products, and process
   B. Activities are individual, and process is important, automatic, and noncortical
   C. Activities are primarily nonverbal, and end products are process-oriented and individual.
   D. Activities are group-oriented, verbal and nonverbal, and process- and product-oriented

647. In the same schematic representation the third level refers to the experience of performing actions that have impact on objects and/or the environment. Which of the following would further guide the selection of activities for this experience level?
   A. Activities may use but are not dependent upon verbal activity, end products, and process
   B. Activities are individual, and process is important, automatic, and noncortical
   C. Activities are primarily nonverbal, and end products are process-oriented and individual.
   D. Activities are group-oriented, verbal and nonverbal, and process- and product-oriented

648. In the same schematic representation the fourth level refers to the coordination of thought, body, and other factors. Which of the following would guide the selection of activities for this experience level?
   A. Activities may use but are not dependent upon verbal activity, end products, and process
   B. Activities are individual, and process is important, automatic, and noncortical
   C. Activities are primarily nonverbal, and end products are process-oriented and individual.
   D. Activities are group-oriented, verbal and nonverbal, and process- and product-oriented

649. In the Rood or neurophysiological approach to treatment, developmental patterns are used to evaluate the person's level of development, which determines the level of treatment. When it is determined to use sensory stimulation for proprioceptors, which of the following should be used?
A. Light touch
B. Ice
C. Slow stroking
D. Vibrations

650. When it is determined to use sensory stimulation for exteroceptive input, which of the following should be used?
A. Light touch
B. Ice
C. Slow stroking
D. Vibrations

651. When it is determined to use an inhibitory procedure in the Rood approach, which of the following should be used?
A. Light touch
B. Ice
C. Slow stroking
D. Vibrations

652. In using the Rood technique of slow stroking, the therapist instructs the student to stroke the person continuously for 4 minutes as part of the therapy. The student corrects the therapist and states, correctly, that slow stroking should not be continued for more than
A. 1 minute
B. 2 minutes
C. 2-1/2 minutes
D. 3 minutes

653. In the Rood technique, depending upon the type of muscle tone and developmental level of the person needing therapy, a treatment program may be
A. all inhibitory and no facilitating
B. inhibitory and facilitating
C. all facilitating
D. all inhibitory, inhibitory and facilitating, all facilitating

654. A therapist introducing proprioceptive neuromuscular facilitation to a new student stated that Kabat, Knott, and Voss developed this therapy system and that current techniques include maximal resistance, postural and righting reflexes, mass movement patterns, reversal of antagonist, and ice. The student suggested that to complete the list the therapist add
   A. vibration
   B. quick stretch
   C. flexion synergies
   D. extension synergies

655. A therapist introducing a student to working with people who have acquired hemiplegia stated that Signe Brunnstrom delineated the stages of recovery and techniques to facilitate recovery. Brunnstrom stated that treatment consists of developing the potential for coordinated movement with reflexlike mechanisms, sensory cues, volitional efforts, and graduation of demand through the six stages of recovery. Which statement about the stages of recovery did the student add to make the information more complete?
   A. The stages follow a definite sequence
   B. The stages can follow any sequence
   C. The stages can skip any stage and plateau anywhere
   D. The stages follow a definite sequence, never skip a stage, and plateau at any one stage

656. In further introducing the student to the treatment process for hemiplegia developed by Brunnstrom the therapist stated that postures and positions used during treatment include supine, sitting, and standing. Volitional effort and functional activities should be initiated early and are considered necessary if there is to be carryover by the person with the problem. The therapist asks "What have I omitted that would make this more complete?" The student answers that
   A. tactile and sensory input are used throughout treatment
   B. visual and verbal clues are used throughout treatment
   C. a total sensory integrated mechanism is used throughout treatment
   D. no other procedures or techniques are used by Brunnstrom

657. In describing the basic idea of orthokinetics to a student a therapist states that a cuff is composed of elastic and inelastic parts. The cuff is placed over those body parts where support and muscle activity are desired. The therapist asks the student which of the following statements is correct.
   A. The elastic or inactive field becomes facilitating
   B. The elastic or active field becomes inhibitory
   C. The inelastic or inactive field becomes inhibitory, and the elastic or active field becomes the facilitator
   D. The cuffs work either way, depending upon which surface is placed on the muscle belly

182 / Occupational Therapy

658. In explaining to an occupational therapy student about the sensory integrative theory constructed by Ayres, the therapist states that the objective of the approach is to enhance the brain's ability to develop the capacity to perceive, remember, and motor plan in order to provide a basis for mastery of all academic and other tasks rather than to focus on specific content. The therapist then asks the student: "Toward what, then, is the therapeutic approach directed?" The student states that
   A. it is directed toward controlling sensory input in order to activate brain mechanisms
   B. it is directed toward integrating sensory input in order to activate brain mechanisms
   C. it is directed toward the development of academic tasks in order to activate brain mechanisms
   D. it is directed toward the development of skill tasks in order to activate brain mechanisms

659. In further explanation to a student of the Ayres concept for treatment, the therapist states that one of the implications for the therapeutic process lies in the premise that some neurons require convergence of many impulses. The therapist then asks the student: "The summation of stimuli directed toward a specific response would be more effective with which of the following?"
   A. Stimuli from one modality directed toward a specific response used frequently
   B. Stimuli from various sensory modalities directed toward a specific response
   C. Stimuli from various sensory modalities directed toward general responses in the area needed
   D. Stimuli from a single sensory modality along with cognitive input at the same time interval

660. In continuing to orient a student to the Ayres concept the therapist states that awareness from action or feedback from the somatosensory and vestibular system is important in organizing and using a sensory input for motor performance. In planning an activity for treatment for a person needing to utilize procedures that emphasize the process of accurate discriminative information the therapist asks the student: "Which activities are most preferable?"
    A. Activities of interest to the person doing them
    B. Complex motor activities creating a challenge
    C. Activities that have simple motor demands
    D. Motor activities requiring a great many responses

661. A person is referred to the occupational therapy service area for self-care activities. The therapist and student visit the person on the ward while the person is still in bed. The student wishes to transfer the person to a chair to do the self-care activities. The therapist suggests that for self-care activities in a chair, the person
    A. needs to be gradually put into a sitting position
    B. needs to be able to maintain trunk balance
    C. should be brought to the service area where all activities are taught
    D. should be taught parallel activities to create motivation

662. A person confined to a bed on a ward is referred to occupational therapy for independent eating. The person indicates his/her need in wishing to eat by himself/herself. The therapist states to the student that independent eating can start as soon as the
    A. person can sit comfortably in a bed or wheelchair or tilted on a tilt board
    B. person is transported to the occupational therapy service area
    C. nurses agree to carry through on the program once it starts
    D. dietary department agrees to let the student have the food to feed the person

663. In working with a person in self-care and/or dressing procedures many basic considerations should be employed. One consideration relative to adaptive equipment is that little or no adaptive equipment should be used unless it is absolutely necessary and then primarily
   A. to motivate the person in showing success
   B. for safety and to reduce energy
   C. to show the person that eating or dressing can be accomplished
   D. to demonstrate the many ways eating or dressing can be accomplished with adaptive equipment.

664. A student is arranging for activities of daily living for a person who has suffered an injury at the C4 level resulting in quadriplegia. The therapist suggests that the student use
   A. zippers, velcro fastenings, plastic cuff, plate guards, and so forth
   B. a 24-hour nursing program
   C. an environmental control system
   D. large-size clothes, large buttons, built-up handles, long-handled combs, a toothbrush, and so forth

665. In training a student in the utilization of splints, the therapist states that the static splint has many uses. In the support of a hand or a joint of a person with arthritis the splint
   A. protects weak muscles from being stretched
   B. is used as a substitute for weak muscles
   C. provides a force to counteract a strong muscle group
   D. immobilizes a joint to prevent movement

666. In additional training of a student on static splints, the therapist states that a splint may be indicated to protect weak muscles from being stretched by
   A. providing the force necessary to counteract a strong muscle group
   B. immobilizing a joint to prevent movement
   C. being used as a substitute for the weak muscles
   D. forcing a joint or bone into correct alignment

667. Additional information given the student by the therapist indicates that corrective splinting can
   A. provide the force necessary to counteract a strong muscle group
   B. immobilize a joint to prevent movement
   C. substitute for weak muscles
   D. force a joint or bone into correct alignment

668. The therapist informs the student that whenever possible, the static splint should hold the forearm or hand in
   A. a comfortable position
   B. an anatomical position
   C. a functional position
   D. a position that allows supination and pronation

669. With respect to the use of splints, the therapist should indicate to the student the precautions that should be taken. One complication to watch for is edema. Another problem that arises with prolonged use of a static splint is that
   A. splints get dirty and need to be cleaned
   B. a joint may become immobile
   C. different parts of the splint may move out of alignment
   D. prolonged pressure on the plastic will cause splitting

670. In the implementation of a program the treatment room provides an atmosphere of activity. Activities are geared toward what is interesting, purposeful, and acceptable to the person concerned. Activities are also geared to
   A. having fun as fun is essential in life
   B. showing their relationship to overall rehabilitation goals
   C. making "things" to show accomplishments
   D. diverting the person away from his/her pathology

671. In implementing a splint for a brain-injured person, the therapist must know that among other occupational therapists (OTs), orthotists, and physical therapists (PTs), splinting is
    A. a generally accepted practice
    B. still a controversial subject
    C. strongly accepted by some and not others
    C. strongly accepted by occupational therapists but not by the others

672. Splinting, if planned appropriately, can do certain things for certain dysfunctions. Which splint is apt to do the most good for the restoration of upper extremity function?
    A. A dynamic splint
    B. An orthokinetic splint
    C. A static cock-up splint
    D. A static forearm hand splint

673. Splinting, if planned appropriately, can do certain things for certain dysfunctions. Which splint is apt to do the most good for strengthening palmar grasp, opposition, and prehension?
    A. A dynamic splint
    B. An orthokinetic splint
    C. A static cock-up splint
    D. A static forearm hand splint

674. Splinting, if planned appropriately, can do certain things for certain dysfunctions. Which splint is apt to do the most good in providing a combination of mobilization and support for relief of pain, increased muscle strength, ROM, and muscle reeducation?
    A. A dynamic splint
    B. An orthokinetic splint
    C. A static cock-up splint
    D. A static forearm hand splint

675. An arm sling is commonly used to support the flaccid arm and prevent subluxation of the shoulder. About which force should the therapist be concerned during the treatment process while the person is using the sling during ambulation?
   A. The earth's gravitational pull on the arm
   B. The strength of forearm muscle groups
   C. The weight of the arm pulling against the shoulder
   D. The total weight of the person jarring the shoulder during walking

676. The arm sling is an easily recognizable means of support for the paralyzed arm. The therapist must be careful not to use a sling that will cause
   A. an increase in shoulder abduction and flexor spasticity
   B. a shoulder disarticulation
   C. shoulder pain and an increase in adductor or flexor spasticity
   D. an increase in shoulder adduction and extension spasticity

677. Vibration is used in treatment when the therapist wishes to
   A. dampen or enhance the vestibulocochlear system
   B. stimulate the sensory ending of the neuromuscular spindle
   C. improve sensory response and increase motor function of flaccid muscles
   D. stimulate individual muscle responses

678. Vestibular therapy is used in treatment when the therapist wishes to
   A. dampen or enhance the vestibulocochlear system
   B. stimulate the sensory ending of the neuromuscular spindle
   C. improve sensory response and increase motor function of flaccid muscles
   D. stimulate individual muscle responses

679. Tactile stimulation is used in treatment when the therapist wishes to
   A. dampen or enhance the vestibulocochlear system
   B. stimulate the sensory ending of the neuromuscular spindle
   C. improve sensory response and increase motor function of flaccid muscles
   D. stimulate individual muscle responses

680. Pressure is used in treatment when the therapist wishes to
   A. dampen or enhance the vestibulocochlear system
   B. stimulate the sensory ending of the neuromuscular spindle
   C. improve sensory response and increase motor function of flaccid muscles
   D. stimulate individual muscle responses

681. A therapist wishing to use thermal stimulation as a method of motor control therapy needs to know that when ice is quickly wiped across the palm of the hand or sole of the feet
   A. a facilitating response will take place
   B. an inhibitory response will take place
   C. a tonic response will take place
   D. a phasic response will take place

682. A therapist wishing to use thermal stimulation as a method of motor control therapy needs to know that when a brief application of ice to the skin over the muscle being treated is applied to the palm of the hand or sole of the feet
   A. a facilitating response will take place
   B. an inhibitory response will take place
   C. a tonic response will take place
   D. a phasic response will take place

683. A therapist wishing to use thermal stimulation as a method of motor control therapy needs to know that application of ice for a few seconds over a muscle will produce
    A. a facilitating response
    B. an inhibitory response
    C. a tonic response
    D. a phasic response

684. A therapist is working with a person who needs to develop a swallowing response. Which method of icing is required?
    A. Swiping the skin just under the nose
    B. Swiping the skin along the borders of the rib cage
    C. Swiping the skin over the sternal notch
    D. Swiping the skin over the muscles in the neck

685. A therapist working with a person who has spastic muscles in the shoulder, usually encountered in people who have hemiplegia, can hold the person's elbow, abduct the arm about 35 to 45 degrees, and gently push and hold the head of the humerus into the glenoid fossa. This action will
    A. relax the muscles and relieve the pain
    B. stimulate the muscles so that a ROM can be completed
    C. inhibit the extrinsic muscles of the hand to start an activity
    D. rebias the muscle spindles to decrease tone in the hand and wrist

686. Occupational therapy for a person with burns may often start in the emergency room. Later in treatment the therapist may not do a ROM or muscle test on the burn site areas. Why would a ROM and muscle test be done on the unaffected body segments?
    A. To prevent contractures and deformity
    B. To develop an information base
    C. To develop rapport with the person during this period
    D. To do planning as part of ongoing therapy

687. In treating the burn-injured person, the therapist must help the person plan for a home program. To encourage and convince the person that a treatment plan involving the use of splints and wearing of pressure garments may continue for a year or more after discharge, the therapist must convey to the client
   A. studies show that only 15% of those who followed this plan needed additional surgery
   B. studies show that only 5% of those who followed this plan needed additional surgery
   C. studies show that only 75% of those who followed this plan needed additional surgery
   D. the ratio of length of time following such a plan to need for surgery is immaterial

688. An occupational therapist working with a young person who has been abused or neglected may use play as a treatment modality. The therapist must realize that in this approach
   A. the setting up of play situations guides the therapy
   B. the child and the play guide the therapy
   C. the therapist and the play guide the therapy
   D. the therapy is guided by the treatment team's goals

689. A therapist using a spatiotemporal adaptation theory for children with developmental disabilities will not that when faced with a stressful situation
   A. the child will use previously acquired patterns to adapt and make use of the stress to move to higher levels of functions
   B. the child will use previously acquired patterns to adapt and not make use of the stress to move to a higher level of function
   C. the child will not use previously acquired patterns to adapt but will stop at this point
   D. the child will use previously acquired patterns and even more primitive levels of functioning to adapt

690. The therapist working with a dysfunctioning child's developmental and adaptive performance using the spatiotemporal adaptation theory knows that
   A. the child's performance is the mirror image of an immature normal child's performance
   B. the child's performance is the same as a normal child's only not as quick or precise
   C. the child's performance is not a mirror image of an immature normal child's
   D. the child's performance is not the same as a normal child's nor will any performance be equal to that of the normal child

691. A therapist is working with an infant who demonstrates neck asymmetry past 4 months of age. Which muscles would the therapist be attempting to develop to correct the asymmetry?
   A. Flexors
   B. Extensors
   C. Adductors
   D. Abductors

692. A therapist working with an infant just past 5 months is attempting to develop back extension and stability to reinforce sitting, standing, and walking. Which action would most likely be strengthened?
   A. Scapula elevation
   B. Scapula adduction
   C. Scapula abduction
   D. Scapula depression

693. In an infant who has cerebral palsy, the anterior pelvic tilt is strong because it is not opposed. The therapist in attempting to block this tile tries to balance this tilt by strengthening which muscle group?
   A. Neck muscles
   B. Shoulder muscles
   C. Abdominal muscles
   D. Hip muscles

694. A therapist working with a child with cerebral palsy may find it more meaningful to refer to a type of muscle tone rather than a diagnostic classification when presenting the child's progress. However, to communicate with others who use a diagnostic classification the therapist would describe muscle tone that fluctuates from low to normal as
    A. ataxia
    B. athetosis
    C. flaccidity
    D. spasticity

695. A therapist working with a child with cerebral palsy may find it more meaningful to refer to a type of muscle tone rather than a diagnostic classification when presenting the child's progress. However, to communicate with others who use a diagnostic classification the therapist would describe muscle tone that is extreme and above normal as
    A. ataxia
    B. athetosis
    C. flaccidity
    D. spasticity

696. A therapist working with a child with cerebral palsy may find it more meaningful to refer to a type of muscle tone rather than a diagnostic classification when presenting the child's progress. However, to communicate with others who use a diagnostic classification the therapist would describe muscle tone that fluctuates from below normal to normal as
    A. ataxia
    B. athetosis
    C. flaccidity
    D. spasticity

697. A therapist working with a child with cerebral palsy may find it more meaningful to refer to a type of muscle tone rather than a diagnostic classification when presenting the child's progress. However, to communicate with others who use a diagnostic classification the therapist would describe muscle tone that is characterized by fluctuating low muscle tone as
   A. ataxia
   B. athetosis
   C. flaccidity
   D. spasticity

698. A therapist working with a child with cerebral palsy must be aware that the child may have as many as ___ additional disorders to deal with.
   A. 1 to 3
   B. 2 to 4
   C. 2 to 7
   D. 5 to 9

699. During treatment and reevaluation the therapist working with a child with cerebral palsy (CP) needs to be aware that
   A. no single evaluative tool defines all the abnormalities seen in CP
   B. specific tools developed by OTs will define all abnormalities seen in CP
   C. specific tools developed by OTs and PTs will define all abnormalities seen in CP
   D. specific tools developed for each diagnostic CP classification will define all abnormalities seen in CP

Explanatory Answers

600. (A) In children with dysfunctions from birth, the younger the child, the greater the potential for treatment, because the central nervous system is still developing and primitive patterns have not been strongly established over a long period of time. (REF. 16, p. 54)

601. (B) For some children with severe damage of long standing, the primitive reflexes may be used for locomotion and may be the child's only means of motor function. (REF. 16, p. 54)

602. (B) A person with dysdiodochokinesia has impaired ability to accomplish alternating movements rapidly and smoothly. (REF. 16, p. 54)

603. (A) A tremor is extreme amount of movement of a part occurring during a voluntary movement and is diminished or absent during rest. (REF. 16, p. 54)

604. (D) A person with dysmetria is unable to control muscle length, resulting in overshooting or pointing past the object that is seen. (REF. 16, p. 55)

605. (C) In decomposition of movement joints are involved in separate movement patterns functioning independently rather than smoothly and in coordination. (REF. 16, p. 55)

606. (B) Chorea or choreoid movements are rapid, jerky, irregular movements involving primarily the face and distal extremities. (REF. 16, p. 55)

607. (D) Nonintention or resting tremor occurs when muscles are at rest and disappears temporarily with voluntary activity. (REF. 16, p. 54)

608. (A) Athetosis or athetoid movements are slow, writhing, twisting, and wormlike movements, involving particularly the neck, face, and extremities. (REF. 16, p. 55)

609. (C) Dystonia (a form of athetosis) occurs when increased muscle tone causes distorted postures of the trunk and extremities. (REF. 16, p. 55)

610. (C) A person who has a violent, forceful, flinging movement of the extremities on one side of the body, particularly involving the proximal musculature, can be described as having hemiballismus or a unilateral chorea. (REF. 16, p. 55)

611. (A) Because of the rheumatoid arthritis disease process, tendons may rupture. Muscle ruptures become evident when a person is asked to flex and extend the metacarpophalangeal joints and the fingers droop. (REF. 16, p. 377)

612. (B) Specific goals for occupational therapy in the treatment of a person with rheumatoid arthritis depend upon the problems and needs of the person. General goals are to maintain or increase mobility of joints and increase strength and to work on each joint daily not to the point of pain but for three or four short periods per day, treating a different joint each time. (REF. 16, p. 380)

613. (D) Warming the hand is beneficial in reducing pain in a person who has rheumatoid arthritis. (REF. 16, p. 380)

614. (D) Passive ROM to just beyond the point of pain may be necessary if the person lacks full active ROM. A paraffin bath may be used to reduce the pain. If pain should persist beyond 3 or 4 hours after therapy, the treatment session should be cut or the joint rested. (REF. 16, p. 380)

615. (D) As soon as a spinal shock subsides, return of motor function begins and continues for approximately 1 year. (REF. 16, p. 386)

616. (D) Once lifesaving procedures have been instituted on people with severe burns, positioning to prevent deformity begins immediately by splinting. (REF. 16, p. 401)

617. (B) Telemetry and electrocardiogram monitoring are fairly new procedures and have more detailed guidelines and methods of evaluating when to stop treatment activities. These services are now being provided in some centers by occupational therapists, physical therapists, and others. (REF. 15, p. 741)

618. (D) In a cardiac rehabilitation program one of the goals should be to decrease the patient's and the family's fears through a process of education to facilitate an understand of what is realistic to expect and to encourage the view that a successful recovery from the injury leads to a relatively normal and productive life. (REF. 15, p. 742)

619. (C) Some patients prefer "pure exercise" to other activities because of the value that is placed on exercise by the general public. (REF. 16, p. 243)

620. (D) Motor analysis of activities may be from biomechanical and/or neurodevelopmental points of view. (REF. 16, p. 244)

621. (B) A biomechanical analysis of activity begins by establishing the exact placement of the selected tools and equipment in relation to the person who is to use them. Only analysis of a specific activity under specific conditions is valid. (REF. 16, p. 244)

622. (A) Electromyography (EMG) equipment is used in the process by which electrical potentials produced by contracting muscles are recorded for study. (REF. 16, p. 245)

623. (A) Neurodevelopmental analysis includes consideration of the developmental and neurophysiological aspects of activity such as observing movements and positions involved in an activity to determine if primitive reflexes are being reinforced or if the move is encouraging desirable righting and equilibrium reactions. (REF. 16, p. 247)

624. (D) An occupational behavior activity analysis would be concerned with developmental levels and the potential of the activity to provide the patient with meaningful opportunities to develop competence and balance within his/her life roles in society. (REF. 15, p. 301)

625. (C) A sensory integrative activity analysis or frame of reference would focus primarily on the sensory, perceptual, and physical aspects of an activity. (REF. 15, p. 297)

626. (C) In using a flat work surface an increase in resistance is needed to give shoulder extension and elbow flexion, and the work surface is inclined down. (REF. 16, p. 249)

627. (B) If the work surface is inclined up, resistance is given to shoulder flexion and elbow extension. (REF. 16, p. 249)

628. (A) If the work surface is raised to the axilla height it will allow flexion and extension of the elbow on a gravity-eliminated plane. (REF. 16, p. 250)

629. (D) If the work surface is lowered to elbow height, supination-pronation movements may be obtained while shoulder rotation is eliminated and the upper arm is allowed to remain adducted. (REF. 16, p. 250)

630. (B) In studies of self-care in patients with chronic illness who regain independence workers hypothesize that the sequence of development reveals an ontogenetic consistency. (REF. 16, p. 464)

631. (A) The sequence followed by chronically ill people who are regaining independence of self-care is feeding, continence, transferring, going to the toilet, dressing, and bathing. (REF. 16, p. 464)

632. (C) The principle of compensation for a limited range of joint motion is to increase the patient's reach by means of extending or enlarging handles. (REF. 16, p. 465)

633. (A) The principle of compensation for incoordination is to provide stability. (REF. 16, p. 470)

634. (B) The principle of compensation for decreased strength is to change body mechanics or techniques or to use lightweight devices or energy-conserving electrical devices. (REF. 16, p. 467)

635. (D) The principle of compensation for the loss of use on one side of the upper extremities is to provide substitutions for the stabilizing or holding function or the involved upper extremity using the assistive or nonpreferred extremity post-CVA. (REF. 16, p. 472)

636. (A) Common architectural design dimensions for the use of a wheelchair in a dwelling should provide 36 inches for the doorway; 30 to 40 inches for the ramp; and approximately 6 degrees or 1 inch to 1 foot for the ramp incline equipped with railings. (REF. 15, p. 245)

637. (C) In normal developmental sequencing a disadvantage is that for handicapped persons the developmental sequence may increase rather than reduce problems. (REF. 18, p. 132)

638. (A) In normal activity sequencing many steps have a logical sequence but may not be necessarily invariant and may require less total time or a repetition of steps. For some handicaps this may be a disadvantage, because the person might do better by splitting up a "normal" sequence. (REF. 18, p. 132)

639. (D) In a task analysis each step in a sequence is examined separately; however, a major drawback is that performance may not occur normally in steps but may be an integrated continuous flow that cannot be broken up. (REF. 18, p. 133)

640. (C) Intervening directly in the pathology of the person and effecting changes or interruptions in that pathology is one of the occupational therapy processes. (REF. 15, p. 302)

641. (A) Maintenance of function refers to the process that must take place when one deals with people who have chronic debilitating or deteriorating conditions. Occupational therapy is then based on strengths and is geared to the promotion of optimum function. (REF. 15, p. 302)

642. (B) The developmental and occupational behavior frame of reference places greater emphasis on building upon the strengths and healthy parts of the person. Therefore it seems to make its major contribution in the area of rehabilitation, maintenance, and prevention. (REF. 15, p. 302)

643. (D) The implementation process has three parts: orientation, development, and termination. (REF. 15, p. 309)

644. (A) Development of an occupational therapy program requires translation of the objectives into specific activities that must be relevant to the objectives and have meaning for the client. (REF. 15, p. 309)

645. (B) At the first level of a schematic representation for a quick guide to the selection of activities for treatment, the process of the activity is important and also automatic and noncortical. The focus of the activity is individual. These enhance the first level called body awareness experience; where movement and sensory input activities are important. (REF. 15, p. 311)

646. (C) At the second level is body effectiveness experience, where one experiences the ability of the body to perform according to some internalized image. Activities here are primarily nonverbal and process-oriented, and their focus is individual. (REF. 15, p. 311)

647. (A) At the third level is the experience of performing actions that have an impact on objects and on the environment. Activities at this level may use (but are not dependent upon) verbal activity, but they are primarily nonverbal end products. Process is important, and the focus is individual and personal. (REF. 15, p. 311)

648. (D) At the fourth level, coordination of thought, body, and other related factors, activities are group-oriented, verbal and nonverbal, and process- and product-oriented. (REF. 15, p. 312)

649. (D) In the Rood technique vibration is used to stimulate the proprioceptors as are rubbing pressure into the muscle belly, joint compression, quick stretch, and appropriate vestibular input. (REF. 15, p. 117)

650. (A) In the Rood technique light touch and/or brushing is used to stimulate the exteroceptive input. Ice, if used at all, is applied with great caution and only to the extremities. (REF. 15, p. 117)

651. (C) Inhibitory procedures used by Rood include slow stroking, neutral warmth, and slow rolling and pressure to the muscle insertion. (REF. 15, p. 117)

652. (D) In the Rood technique slow stroking is done for no more than 3 minutes. (REF. 15, p. 117)

653. (D) Depending upon the type of muscle tone and the developmental level of the person, a treatment program may be all inhibitory, inhibitory and facilitating, or all facilitating. (REF. 15, p. 117)

654. (B) Current techniques used in proprioceptive neuromuscular facilitation are quick stretch, maximal but not overpowering resistance, postural and righting reflexes, mass movement patterns with spiral and diagonal components, reversal of antagonist, and application of ice. (REF. 15, p. 118)

655. (D) The stages of recovery stated by Brunnstrom follow a definite sequence, and the person never skips a stage; however, a person may plateau at one of the six stages. (REF. 15, p. 118)

656. (B) In the Brunnstrom techniques visual and verbal clues are used throughout treatment, along with postures, positions, and volitional effort. Functional activities are initiated early in order to create carryover by the person with the problem. (REF. 15, p. 119)

657. (D) The basic idea in orthokinetics is the use of a cuff made of elastic and inelastic parts. The elastic or active field covers those parts where muscle activity is desired. The inactive field thus becomes the inhibitory field, and the active field becomes the facilitating field. (REF. 15, p. 119)

658. (A) The therapeutic approach in the Ayres theory is directed toward controlling sensory input in order to activate brain mechanisms. (REF. 15, p. 123)

659. (B) The convergence of sensory input indicates that the therapeutic process lies in the premise that some neurons require convergence of many impulses for discharge. Thus, the summation of stimuli from various sensory modalities, when directed toward a specific response, may be more effective than input from one modality alone. (REF. 15, p. 123)

660. (C) Activities that have simple motor demands and require integrative responses are preferable to more complex motor activities requiring a great many responses that cannot be adequately integrated. They are utilized when activities are needed to emphasize the processing of accurate discriminative information. (REF. 15, p. 124)

661. (B) Once trunk balance can be maintained, a person may proceed with self-care activities in a chair. (REF. 15, p. 231)

662. (A) Independent eating may be started as soon as a person can sit comfortably in bed or in a wheelchair; in some instances, it may be started while the person is tilted on a tilt bed or a tilt board. (REF. 15, p. 231)

663. (B) In self-care and dressing one basic consideration relative to adaptive equipment is that little or no adaptive equipment should be used unless it is absolutely necessary and then primarily for safety and/or to reduce energy and save time. (REF. 15, p. 232)

664. (C) In the case of a person with a C4 injury resulting in quadriplegia, sophisticated environmental control systems can be recommended, because function at this level is limited. (REF. 15, p. 236)

665. (B) A static splint can support the hand, joint, or arch as a substitute for weak muscles in people with arthritis. (REF. 15, p. 454)

666. (A) A static splint may be indicated to protect weak muscles from being stretched by providing the force to counteract a strong muscle group. (REF. 15, p. 454)

667. (D) A corrective splint can specifically position or force an involved joint or a bone into correct or near-correct alignment. (REF. 15, p. 454)

668. (C) Static splints have no movable parts and, whenever possible, should hold the involved forearm and hand in a functional position. (REF. 15, p. 454)

669. (B) The therapist should be aware that static splints can cause swelling and edema. Prolonged static splinting can cause immobility of joints. (REF. 15, p. 454)

670. (B) Activity not only is geared toward what is interesting, purposeful, and acceptable but also is geared so that the person in treatment can see its relevance to its overall rehabilitative goals. (REF. 15, p. 377)

671. (B) Splinting for the brain-injured person remains a controversial subject among physicians, OTs, orthotists, and PTs. This controversy is caused by the variety of treatment approaches and settings available. (REF. 15, p. 386)

672. (C) A static cock-up splint, when planned appropriately, may be beneficial in the restoration of upper extremity function as it would support the weak wrist in a functional position both at rest and during activity of the entire extremity. (REF. 15, p. 386-387)

673. (A) A dynamic splint using the long opponens with an outrigger system and finger cuffs would encourage active use of the fingers during resistive functional exercises to strengthen palmar grasp, opposition, and prehension. (REF. 15, p. 387)

674. (B) An orthokinetic splint provides a combination of mobilization and support and can be used for relief of pain, increase of muscle strength, ROM, and muscle reeducation. (REF. 15, p. 387)

675. (A) An arm sling is commonly used both to support the flaccid areas and to prevent subluxation of the shoulder caused by excess gravitational pull on weak muscles during ambulation. (REF. 15, p. 387)

676. (C) The arm sling is an easily recognized means of support for the paralyzed. Care must be taken not to use a sling that well cause shoulder pain, an increase in adductor or flexor spasticity, or shoulder subluxation, all of which are the results of poor design, application, use, and/or monitoring. (REF. 15, p. 387)

677. (B) At the present time, it appears that the primary sensory ending of the neuromuscular spindle is highly sensitive to vibration, which is why vibrators are used in treatment. (REF. 15, p. 112)

678. (A) The connections and pathways of the vestibulocochlear system are many and intricate. Stimulation of either the vestibular or cochlear system will enhance the other. Basically any movement done slowly and repeatedly will dampen the system, while rapid movement will enhance it. (REF. 15, p. 112)

679. (C) Application of stimuli to the skin over flaccid muscles, using touch and moderate pressure, can result in improved sensory response and increased motor function. (REF. 15, p. 385)

680. (D) Pressure over a muscle belly, joint, or tendon will stimulate individual muscle response. (REF. 15, p. 385)

681. (D) A quick application of ice on the palm or sole will produce a phasic response. (REF. 16, p. 65)

682. (A) The brief application of ice to the skin over the muscle being treated or rubbing of ice over the palm or sole is facilitating in nature. (REF. 16, p. 65)

683. (C) A tonic response is obtained when ice is maintained over a muscle for a few seconds. (REF. 16, p. 65)

684. (C) Swallowing can be initiated by swiping ice over the skin at the sternal notch. (REF. 16, p. 65)

685. (A) Joint approximation or light joint compression is used to inhibit spastic muscles, relieve pain, and relax muscles. To relieve pain from spastic muscles of the shoulder the person's elbow is held, the arm is abducted to 35-45 degrees, and the head of the humerus is gently pushed into and held in the glenoid fossa. (REF. 16, p. 77)

686. (B) Although occupational therapists may treat people who have had severe burns upon emergency admission, later in therapy ROM and muscle testing of the burn site may be too painful. However, the therapist can evaluate unaffected body segments as a comparison and develop an information base for further treatment when the area heals. (REF. 16, p. 403)

687. (A) A therapist can encourage and convince a person and/or his or her family that when splints and pressurized garments are prescribed for home care, only 15% of the people who follow this regimen for a year or more need additional surgery as compared with 70% needing surgery who failed the program for 6 months. (REF. 16, p. 407)

688. (B) Treatment of young children who have been abused is complicated. Using play as a medium in therapy requires the therapist to shift roles from "directing" an activity to participating in the activity. The therapist sets up situations for treatment goals, but it is the child and the play itself that guides the therapy. (REF. 20, p. 319)

689. (B) The spatiotemporal adaptation therapy addresses some problems in adaptation under stress. Generally there is a similarity between patterns used by normal children during developmental phases and patterns used by children with developmental dysfunctions. Under stress normal children will use previously acquired patterns to adapt but will make use of the stress to move to higher levels of development. Children with dysfunctions are able to make use of the stress to move to higher levels of function and may continue to perform at primitive levels or continue to attempt higher level activities by using lower level functions. (REF. 15, p. 562)

690. (C) Although a dysfunctioning child's developmental and adaptive performances seem to reflect patterns used by normal children at less mature stages, the dysfunctioning child's performance is not a mirror image of an immature normal child's performance. (REF. 15, p. 564)

691. (A) Neck asymmetry is normally seen in infants until the age of 3 to 4 months when flexors or muscles develop, bring the head to midline, and allow symmetry to develop. (REF. 15, p. 646)

692. (B) In normal development, scapula adduction reinforces back extension and stability. It is normal in 4- and 6-month-old infants in a prone suspension. If this action does not occur, primitive and abnormal development may result. (REF. 15, p. 647)

693. (C) The anterior pelvic tilt or lordosis is seen in the prone 4-month-old infant. When the infant reaches 4 to 5 months of age the anterior pelvic tilt is balanced by the abdominal muscles. Later, the abdominals and the hip extension work together to balance the anterior pelvic tilt. (REF. 15, p. 647)

694. (B) An individual with pure athetosis has muscle tone that fluctuates from low to normal. (REF. 15, p. 649)

695. (D) Spasticity refers to extreme and above-normal muscle tone. (REF. 15, p. 648)

696. (A) Ataxia refers to muscle tone that fluctuates from below normal to normal. (REF. 15, p. 650)

697. (C) Flaccidity is characterized by fluctuating low muscle tone. (REF. 15, p. 650)

698. (C) Studies have shown that most children with cerebral palsy have anywhere from two to seven additional disorders. The following are estimates of percentages of other disorders: 50% vision, 25% auditory, 25% speech, 14% sensory integrative disor-

ders, 50 to 75% below-average intelligence, 25% seizures. Emotional problems are common. (REF. 15, p. 651)

699. (A) OTs should be aware that there is no single evaluation tool that defines the many abnormalities seen in the child with cerebral palsy; however, there are many tools that can be used in conjunction with each other to result in a more accurate evaluation. (REF. 15, p. 651)

9 Management/ Administration

QUESTIONS 701–711: Select the **one** most appropriate answer.

700. The American Occupational Therapy Association (AOTA) was formerly the National Society for the Promotion of Occupational Therapy, Inc. In which year was the society founded?
 A. 1914
 B. 1917
 C. 1920
 D. 1923

701. In which year did the society change its name to the American Occupational Therapy Association:
 A. 1914
 B. 1917
 C. 1920
 D. 1923

702. The first occupational therapists to become registered did so in the year
 A. 1920
 B. 1923
 C. 1931
 D. 1948

208 / Occupational Therapy

703. The first advanced master's degree program for occupational therapists, registered, (OTRs) began in the year
   A. 1920
   B. 1923
   C. 1931
   D. 1948

704. The AOTA began a program of approving educational programs for occupational therapy assistants in the year
   A. 1931
   B. 1948
   C. 1959
   D. 1965

705. AOTA history includes the formation of the American Occupational Therapy Foundation (AOTF). In which year was it founded?
   A. 1931
   B. 1948
   C. 1959
   D. 1965

706. The AOTA's general purpose in furtherance of its objectives as set forth in its Articles of Incorporation is
   A. to act as a charitable, scientific, literary, and educational organization
   B. to act as an advocate for occupational therapy in education, research, action, service, and standards
   C. to establish essentials and, thus, to establish occupational therapy curricula
   D. to establish and enforce standards of practice

707. The general purpose of the American Occupational Therapy Foundation is
   A. to act as a charitable, scientific, literary, and educational organization
   B. to act as an advocate for occupational therapy in education, research, action, service, and standards
   C. to establish essentials and, thus, to establish occupational therapy curricula
   D. to establish and enforce standards of practice

708. The AOTA Representative Assembly (formerly the Delegate Assembly) is
   A. a forum for each state to share occupational therapy concerns
   B. a group of members from each state who discuss occupational therapy concerns
   C. the legislative and policymaking body
   D. the standards and enforcement body of the association

709. In addition to representatives from the District of Columbia and Puerto Rico, the AOTA Representative Assembly includes
   A. one representative from each state
   B. one representative from each state that has a state association
   C. proportional representation from each state
   D. proportional representation relative to the U.S. Congress from each state

710. The AOTA Representative assembly is presided over by the
   A. president of AOTA
   B. vice-president of AOTA
   C. president of AOTA's Representative Assembly
   D. speaker of AOTA's Representative Assembly

711. Officers of the AOTA Representative Assembly are elected by the
   A. Representative Assembly's own members
   B. AOTA membership
   C. officers of the AOTA
   D. officers of the AOTA's Representative Assembly

QUESTIONS 712–714: The AOTA Representative Assembly has three commissions: Standards and Ethics, Education, and Practice. Each commission is chaired by an individual who is either recommended or elected and is then confirmed or ratified by the Representative Assembly.

712. The chair of the Commission on Standards and Ethics is
    A. recommended by the AOTA president
    B. recommended by the head of the Representative Assembly
    C. elected by its own members
    D. elected by AOTA members

713. The chair of the Commission on Education is
    A. recommended by the AOTA president
    B. recommended by the head of the Representative Assembly
    C. elected by its own members
    D. elected by AOTA members

714. The chair of the Commission on Practice is
    A. recommended by the AOTA president
    B. recommended by the head of the Representative Assembly
    C. elected by its own members
    D. elected by AOTA members

QUESTIONS 715–723: Select the **one** most appropriate answer.

715. The Accreditation Committee's function is the accreditation or approval
    A. of certification of the OTR
    B. of educational programs
    C. of the standards of practice
    D. of the reviews of the format and content of standards

716. The AOTA Executive Board is composed of
    A. no paid members
    B. all paid members
    C. only one paid member
    D. all paid members except one

717. The Executive Board is responsible for
    A. implementation of the association's policies
    B. implementation of the business of the Representative Assembly
    C. management of the Representative Assembly
    D. management of the association

718. The national office of the AOTA is responsible for
    A. implementation of the association's policies
    B. implementation of the business of the Representative Assembly
    C. management of the Representative Assembly
    D. management of the association

719. The executive director of the AOTA is
    A. the same person as the president
    B. elected by the members
    C. appointed by the president
    D. employed by the association

720. The executive director of the AOTA
    A. manages the operations of the national office
    B. is the manager of the Representative Assembly
    C. is the chief executive officer of the association
    D. discharges presidential duties in the absence of the president

721. The World Federation of Occupational Therapists (WFOT) is
    A. composed of OTRs who work overseas
    B. composed of people interested in occupational therapy overseas
    C. a formal organization like AOTA
    D. a part of the AOTA

212 / Occupational Therapy

722. AOTA offers a wide range of benefits to its members.
  A. These benefits are free to all members
  B. These benefits are free to all members but not to the public
  C. Some benefits are free but other are charged
  D. These benefits are free to members and charged to those who are certified only

723. A person who successfully passes the certification examination for Occupational Therapist, Registered, must pay which of the following to become an OTR and a member of AOTA?
  A. Payment of one fee
  B. One fee for certification and one fee for membership
  C. An examination fee
  D. A certification fee

QUESTIONS 724–727: The association confers on members and friends of the profession a number of different awards or certificates. Match the award with its description.

  A. given to OTRs in recognition of significant contributions
  B. the highest honor of the association
  C. given to Certified Occupational Therapy Assistants (COTAs) in recognition of significant contributions
  D. the highest academic honor of the association

724. Award of Merit
725. Eleanor Clarke Slagle Lectureship
726. Roster of Fellows
727. Roster of Honors

Management/Administration / 213

QUESTIONS 728–732: Select the **one** most appropriate answer.

728. To direct, govern, and legislate itself and its members the AOTA has developed
 A. bylaws and a constitution
 B. bylaws only
 C. a constitution only
 D. parliamentary rules and procedures from *Roberts Rules of Order, Newly Revised*

729. An individual AOTA member in good standing is one who, among other things, has
 A. paid his or her fee
 B. passed the certification examination
 C. a special interest in occupational therapy
 D. made significant contributions to the field

730. The AOTA has developed "essentials" for occupational therapy curricula. Which statement is true?
 A. These essentials are the same for OTRs and COTAs
 B. These essentials are completely different for OTRs and COTAs
 C. Half of the essentials are for OTRs and the other half for COTAs
 D. The same essentials are used for both OTRs and COTAs with subsections for each

731. The OTR must pass a certification examination offered by the AOTA. This is
 A. the same examination given to COTAs
 B. completely different from the examination given to COTAs
 C. in part the same examination given to COTAs
 D. the same examination given to COTAs but a different passing score is used

732. The status of licensure has become a reality in many states, the District of Columbia, and Puerto Rico. In which year did the first licensure for occupational therapy take place?
   A. 1951
   B. 1961
   C. 1971
   D. 1976

QUESTIONS 733–737: Preparation of a budget may generally involve the items listed below unless a specific state or agency has set rates.

---

733. When preparing an occupational therapy budget, the occupational therapy administrator should be aware that
   A. the indirect costs and direct costs are 50-50
   B. the indirect costs are higher than the direct costs
   C. the direct costs are higher than the indirect costs
   D. the hospital administrator takes care of the indirect costs

734. Considering a 40% indirect cost, the amount for a $130,400 direct-cost occupational therapy budget would be
   A. $48,933
   B. $56,933
   C. $86,933
   D. $99,933

735. In determining an occupational therapy budget, the supervisor should consider
   A. direct costs
   B. direct and indirect costs
   C. direct and indirect costs and bad debt allowance
   D. direct and indirect costs and faculty education

736. In determining the fee for service the total budget is divided by the
    A. number of patients to be seen
    B. number of procedures to be performed
    C. number of days and therapists one uses
    D. amount of money one wishes to make

737. To plan a controlled budget for a budget period in addition to monitoring the results the occupational therapy administrator must divide the budget by the
    A. number of months
    B. number of projected procedures
    C. number of therapists on staff
    D. total number of people on staff

QUESTIONS 738–800: Select the **one** most appropriate answer.

738. A management report must be understood at many levels. To do this the administrative therapist should
    A. write in simple English and short sentences
    B. write progress reports
    C. write in a style accepted within the facility's system
    D. write in descriptive yet short reports

739. Research in occupational therapy is
    A. in its infancy
    B. well established
    C. done only in conjunction with other disciplines
    D. not necessary

740. Much of the research in occupational therapy completed thus far
    A. supports occupational therapy theory
    B. is descriptive of client characteristics
    C. is of little value
    D. does not need to be pursued

741. Within the medical community the
    A. terms "referral" and "prescription" are used incorrectly
    B. terms "referral" and "prescription" often are used interchangeably
    C. term "referral" is the only one used
    D. term "prescription" is old and "referral" is the new term

742. When occupational therapy is offered as part of a medical management program, a referral or a prescription must be signed by a physician. In fact, daily practice suggests that
    A. the referral is most highly considered
    B. the prescription is passé
    C. both are passé
    D. both are current

743. To evaluate and select goals for occupational therapy most physicians
    A. are not knowledgeable enough about occupational therapy
    B. do not care enough about occupational therapy to bother
    C. do not know enough about occupational therapy goals, so they do not send patients
    D. leave goal selection entirely up to the OTR without concern

744. If a physician has inadequate education in rehabilitation services, it is up to the
    A. physician to obtain this information
    B. physician's school to give this information
    C. physical medicine and rehabilitation or other departments to give this information to the physician
    D. occupational therapists to educate the physician

745. If physicians know a lot about occupational therapy, their role then is
    A. to coordinate and manage patient services
    B. to coordinate and manage occupational therapy services
    C. to coordinate and manage the OTRs who serve their patients
    D. to let the occupational therapy service carry on without them

746. Referrals from nurses, speech pathologists, social workers, and others may
    A. be received and acted on
    B. be received and turned over to the physician
    C. not be received
    D. be received only if they work in the same institution

747. In the evaluation of a referral from a source other than a physician the OTR should
    A. proceed with whatever treatment is necessary
    B. proceed with treatment only if the source is within the same facility
    C. determine if medical management is necessary and receive it
    D. determine what she/he can do and do it but not charge for it

748. Provided no third-party payment is to be processed, a physician's consent may not be necessary when a referral comes to occupational therapy for developing a
    A. health maintenance or prevention program
    B. long-range goal for posthospital care
    C. very short-range goal for an inpatient
    D. long-range goal for an outpatient

749. Occupational therapists themselves may refer individuals
    A. only to others in the same facility
    B. only to other OTRs
    C. to any agency, facility, or professional
    D. to any agency approved by their facility

218 / Occupational Therapy

750. In some medical management programs, especially mental health, referrals to occupational therapy may be routine and are sometimes called "blanket referrals." These referrals pose
   A. no problems and allow the OTR free rein
   B. some problems in that the physician may be unaware of the OTR's goals and objectives for the patient
   C. no problems because the goals and objectives are established for the occupational therapy department
   D. some problems because OTRs do not stay in mental health work for long periods

751. With respect to the blanket referral, occupational therapists should
   A. encourage it because it brings in more patients who bring in more money
   B. discourage it because it is unprofessional
   C. encourage it as a way of increasing the size of staff
   D. discourage it as a device to use occupational therapy as a diversional or recreational program

752. Certification of a COTA is granted by
   A. the AOTA
   B. the AOTA and the AMA
   C. COTA's own association
   D. an ad hoc American OT Certification Board

753. Management of an occupational therapy department differs little from the management of other health care groups. The range of problems facing any manager regardless of discipline is
   A. controlled by the manager, thus reducing management to a functional level
   B. so great that one habitual set of responses or alternatives by a manager is inadequate
   C. restricted by the manager in order to motivate his/her staff to accomplish their goals
   D. reduced by discipline, thus allowing the manager to be able to handle all problems through his/her own style

Management/Administration / 219

754. Reed and Sanderson list eight basic performance criteria each occupational therapist should be able to enact. Continuing education is one of these. Occupational therapists should participate in continuing education because
   A. they need it for licensure
   B. universities cannot teach new therapists all the information they need to know
   C. hospitals, agencies, and institutions pay for it, so it is free
   D. staff promotions are dependent on it

755. Continuing education is needed by therapists because
   A. information is constantly increasing, changing, and being revised and continuing education is a way to receive new information
   B. it is required for licensure
   C. staff promotions are dependent upon it
   D. it is the fastest growing education program in the country and OTRs should be a part of it

756. One of the relatively recent additions to the health care lexicon is "quality assurance." Which best describes quality assurance?
   A. Concern for monitoring and evaluating the quality and appropriateness of patient care
   B. Concern that the hospital/agency prohibits discrimination and has established quality guidelines for testing and selection procedures for all health care personnel
   C. Concern that credentialing, licensure, and practice standards or protocols are regulated to assure or improve quality of care
   D. Concern and purpose in showing what has happened to the person during treatment, including the cost containment factor

757. Studies have shown that successful managers use participative management. The building of consensus is one element of this approach wherein the staff must come to a consensus on what the real problems are and how they will solve them. This approach is
   A. almost impossible to achieve
   B. simple but time consuming
   C. complex but effective
   D. easy for a strong manager

758. Certification and licensure for OTRs are
   A. identical
   B. identical only in certain states
   C. granted by the same agency
   D. granted by a nongovernment agency (certification) and a government agency (licensure)

759. Record keeping is an ongoing function in any service. Carefully kept records may
   A. document the course of intervention
   B. be a way for administrators to keep track of therapists
   C. keep staff from duplicating services
   D. show a well-organized occupational therapy department

760. In most cases the format for record keeping is
   A. outlined by the occupational therapy manager
   B. agreed upon by consensus in the occupational therapy department
   C. outlined by regulations for and by the institution
   D. agreed upon by the top manager of the institution

761. Record keeping should above all else
   A. include mainly subjective feelings
   B. contain mainly objective facts
   C. contain some objective feelings and some objective facts
   D. include objective facts and subjective feelings based on objective facts

762. In record keeping the most desirable practice is to
    A. use facts that can be measured to the maximum
    B. use any fact as long as the information is covered
    C. utilize any information heard, seen, or experienced
    D. utilize only the data heard, seen, or experienced

763. In discharge planning, prevention of further injury or illness involves knowledge of many safety factors plus professional knowledge about the person's progress. Such a combination of knowledge
    A. ensures that the therapist takes whatever action is necessary to communicate these factors to the person with the illness and to others on the team
    B. should be possessed, but the responsibility belongs to the physician to disseminate this information
    C. is found in the team members, and each takes responsibility accordingly
    D. is important; however, institutional or hospital policy dictates what each team person is to do

764. For occupational therapists to implement occupational therapy services in today's complex environment they must have a system. One system suggested is the General Systems Theory. The main objective of this approach is to provide a framework for
    A. communication within the occupational therapy service
    B. communication between specialists
    C. satisfying third-party payees
    D. satisfying specific occupational therapy procedures

765. General Systems Theory is used to describe a level of theoretical model building. Which statement closely describes this model?
    A. It introduces arbitrary techniques to analyze the relationship of the parts to the whole
    B. It uses a mathematical approach to examine the relationship of the parts to the whole
    C. It accepts the complexities of the system and searches for a structural pattern to examine the parts and the whole
    D. It uses a specific scientific approach to examine the parts and the whole

766. A problem of the system's approach is that it
    A. lacks clarity
    B. seems so clear that no one believes it will work
    C. often goes counter to the agency's general system
    D. is only a theory

767. The skill gained from a systems approach assists the occupational therapy manager and individual clinician in gaining
    A. authority
    B. power
    C. recognition
    D. status

768. A manager with power has more opportunity than one without power to
    A. maintain control over activities within his/her jurisdiction
    B. be more creative and explore
    C. give commands and take action
    D. run a shipshape organization

769. One of the management tools used by an occupational therapy director to establish programs is
    A. staff attitudes and concerns
    B. staff consensus
    C. current trends in treatment
    D. budget

770. When staffing functions are established the occupational therapy manager must require
   A. that both the quality and/or number of persons necessary to accomplish the objectives be identified
   B. that only the quality of work necessary to accomplish the objectives be obtained
   C. a generous budget to attract the necessary therapist to accomplish objectives
   D. an adequate budget to hire a staff in keeping with the size of the other support services offered

771. In the hiring of an occupational therapist a job specification is prepared on the basis of the job description. The job specification
   A. identifies maximum acceptable qualifications
   B. identifies minimum acceptable qualifications
   C. is a general guide to job duties including salary
   D. is a specific guide to job duties including salary

772. The federal government's Privacy Act of 1974 limits the information that can be obtained in a reference check on a prospective employee to
   A. education, character, and work performance
   B. grade point average (GPA), school activities, and clinical experience
   C. actual employment, time spent on the job, and salary
   D. supervisory reports, promotions if any, and quality of work

773. During the actual interview process, in today's market of supply and demand, which of the following would be a critical point for the employer to ask the prospective occupational therapist?
   A. If the starting salary is fair and commensurate with the employee's experience
   B. If the working conditions offered to the employee are satisfactory
   C. If the employee's job expectations can be met on the job
   D. If the employee can do the job expected in the organization

224 / Occupational Therapy

774. With which of the following sets of conditions would a new employee be more apt at performing all the job functions as described in the job description after the initial probationary period:
   A. Graduation from an excellent school with a high GPA
   B. Good recruitment, sound interview, and good induction to the job by the organization
   C. High score and excellent recommendations from all field work centers
   D. Good working facilities and good educational and field work experience

775. The purpose of a person's medical record is to document the course of that person's health care. The person must be assured that information shared must remain confidential. During which procedure might a person have no say as to where and how this record is used?
   A. Clinical staff meetings
   B. Clinical teaching meetings
   C. Litigation
   D. Decisions requiring reimbursement claims

776. The medical record includes information about an individual's course of treatment collected from many people and departments. The occupational therapy record-keeping procedures may follow:
   A. the one planned by the occupational therapy department
   B. the one planned by the rehabilitation department
   C. any plan by the occupational therapist providing it is accurate and concise
   D. only the plan of the medical records department

777. The "problem-oriented" record is one way to keep patient records. The process for recording in this system is called
   A. PORR -- Problem-Oriented Record Report
   B. SOAP -- Subject-Objective Assessment Plan
   C. SOPR -- Standard Operating Procedure Report
   D. OTSCCRS -- Occupational Therapy Sequential Client Care Recording System

778. Professionals in health care facilities work under a code of ethics. The purpose of such a code is to describe the relationships among the practitioner, the client, and
   A. society
   B. the hospital
   C. the immediate occupational therapy department
   D. the occupational therapy department and the institution/agency

779. AOTA has established Principles of Occupational Therapy Ethics. These principles are intended as a guide for conduct of its members. Therefore, these principles or ethics should
   A. be considered separately from the law
   B. not be considered separately from the law
   C. be considered only when members are "on duty"
   D. be considered only when members are performing certain professional functions

780. The Principles of Occupational Therapy Ethics were intended to be
   A. used in national legislation
   B. used in licensing laws
   C. guiding and preventive rather than negative or disciplinary
   D. used as a definition for clients for standards of care

781. The Principles of Occupational Therapy Ethics were intended to be used
   A. by the national government
   B. by the state government
   C. by the occupational therapy district
   D. only internally by AOTA

782. The AOTA code of ethics states that occupational therapists shall function with discretion and integrity in relations with other professional members. If one becomes aware of objective evidence of a breach of ethics or substandard service the therapist should
   A. talk to the person involved to correct the problem
   B. talk to the person's supervisor and let him/her take action
   C. talk it over with one's immediate supervisor and let him/her take action
   D. take whatever action is necessary according to established procedures

783. Strategic planning is a part of all health care agencies. When an occupational therapy department fails to become involved in such planning
   A. the department will lose value to its organization and will ultimately be eliminated
   B. the department will not lose value as occupational therapists still have not met the supply needed
   C. the department would only lose if the entire agency lost because such departments generally do not make money
   D. the department is part of a rehabilitation service that is needed and will always be used

784. In the developmental portion of any strategic plan adjustments are made to accommodate change. Without access to this phase of planning an occupational therapy director
   A. will look to administration for any support needed
   B. would not need to worry as nationally occupational therapy will always be supported
   C. would find that decisions about the department would be little more than arbitrary
   D. would miss little as most plans last only a few years and everything would change in that time

785. In strategic planning the occupational therapy manager might ask himself/herself the following question about a specific service offered by the department: "If I were not already offering this service, would I do so now?" If the answer is "no" then the manager would
   A. abandon the service
   B. continue the service
   C. reduce the rate (of cost) of that service
   D. increase the rate (of cost) of that service

786. Most if not all occupational therapists are concerned about quality of care for their clients. In this respect, quality assurance is best described as
   A. accreditation of schools, certification of therapists, and licensure of therapists
   B. objective standards for service delivery to clients
   C. assessment of actual service delivery and outcome
   D. recruitment of high-caliber students, high GPAs and field work performance reports

787. In attempting to develop research in occupational therapy it has been said that theories consist of statements that relate concepts. Concepts are a way of classifying the world according to some criteria. Occupational therapy concepts often
   A. are easily defined conceptually
   B. are unclearly defined conceptually
   C. are easily agreed upon by many
   D. have definite operational definitions

788. With respect to the knowledge of occupational therapy that can be developed and tested
   A. very few theories exist
   B. many theories exist
   C. most theories are based upon clinical evidence and have already been tested
   D. most theories are based on clinical data from other disciplines and transfer easily to occupational therapy

789. Occupational therapy practice, for the most part, is based upon
    A. past clinical evidence of successful cases
    B. tradition and untested hypotheses
    C. carefully recorded data from previous cases
    D. theories based upon clinical evidence

790. The *American Journal of Occupational Therapy* made two surveys, in 1973 and 1979, of papers published about occupational therapy. The percentage papers that were research papers
    A. was approximately the same for both years
    B. increased greatly in 1979 compared with 1973
    C. decreased somewhat in 1979 compared with 1973
    D. decreased greatly in 1979 compared with 1973

791. Much of the research in occupational therapy done thus far is
    A. philosophical
    B. experimental
    C. descriptive
    D. scientific

792. The current state of research in occupational therapy represents
    A. political and economic pressures from within and from outside the profession
    B. pressure from the academic side of the profession
    C. pressure from the clinical side of the profession
    D. a process of normal evolution of professional knowledge

793. In the development and/or management of a rehabilitation service, a manager must recognize the interrelated nature of people's varied needs. To meet these needs a manager must make role assignments to departments based on the
   A. traditional role of a discipline
   B. modality used by the discipline
   C. discipline's and/or individual staff's preparation to provide the service
   D. the discipline's facilities and space provided for the modality

794. An occupational therapy manager in establishing staffing patterns and ratios of staff to patients will depend mainly on the
   A. nature of the patient population and organizational structure of the center
   B. standard ratios of other comparable departments in a center
   C. established budget set by the center
   D. standard ratio set by the AOTA

795. A manager in establishing particular roles and duties assigned to staff as well as considering other unique factors in a given center will influence how staffing ratios are set. Ideally, nonsupervisory staff should spend what percent of their time in direct patient care and what percent in support service?
   A. 50%-50%
   B. 60%-40%
   C. 70%-30%
   D. 80%-20%

796. In a psychiatric occupational therapy staff which ratio of staff to patients is suggested?
   A. 1 OTR to 17 patients
   B. 1 OTR to 22 patients
   C. 1 OTR to 27 patients
   D. 1 OTR to 32 patients

797. COTAs could make up part of the occupational therapy staff discussed in Questions 796. Which ratio of OTRs to COTAs is suggested?
   A. 1 OTR to 1 COTA
   B. 1 OTR to 2 COTAs
   C. 1 OTR to 3 COTAs
   D. 1 OTR to 4 COTAs

798. In the organizational structure of rehabilitation services there is continuous debate about the relative merits of a decentralized hospital versus a centralized model. Administrative staff most frequently support a
   A. centralized system
   B. decentralized system
   C. relative balance between the two
   D. straight-line authority system

799. With reference to Question 798, the staff for professional services usually favor a
   A. centralized system
   B. decentralized system
   C. relative balance between the two
   D. straight-line authority system

800. A manager in a new system who wishes to do program planning and development will first address
   A. what changes must be made
   B. who the people available to make changes are
   C. why the changes are necessary
   D. what the service system should look like

Explanatory Answers

700. (B) The National Society for the Promotion of Occupational Therapy was founded in 1917. (REF. 15, p. 9)

701. (D) The society changed its name to AOTA in 1923 (REF. 15, p. 9)

702. (C) The first occupational therapists to become OTRs did so in 1931. (REF. 15, p. 12)

703. (D) The first master's degree program for OTRs started at New York University in 1948. (REF. 9, p. A-1)

704. (C) In 1959 the AOTA began a program of approving educational programs for COTAs. (REF. 9, p. A-2)

705. (D) The AOTF was founded in 1965. (REF. 15, p. 9)

706. (B) The purpose of AOTA, as stated in its incorporation papers, is to act as an advocate for occupational therapy in education, research, action, service, and standards. (REF. 23, p. 7)

707. (A) The purpose of the AOTF is to act as a charitable, scientific, literary, and educational organization. (REF. 15, p. 17)

708. (C) The AOTA Representative Assembly is its legislative and policymaking body. (REF. 23, p. 8)

709. (C) The AOTA Representative Assembly has proportional representation from each state, the District of Columbia, and Puerto Rico. (REF. 23, p. 8)

710. (D) The AOTA Representative Assembly is presided over by its own speaker. (REF. 23, p. 8)

711. (A) Officers of the AOTA Representative Assembly are elected by the Assembly's own members. (REF. 23, p. 8)

712. (A) The chair of the Standards and Ethics Commission is recommended by the AOTA president and ratified by the Representative Assembly. (REF. 9, p. A-5)

713. (C) The chair of the Commission on Education is elected by its own members and ratified by the Representative Assembly. (REF. 9, p. A-5)

714. (A) The chair of the Commission on Practice is recommended by the AOTA president and ratified by the Representative Assembly. (REF. 9, p. A-5)

715. (B) The Accreditation Committee's function is to accredit and approve educational programs. (REF. 9, p. A-6)

716. (C) The executive director of the AOTA, a nonvoting member of the Executive Board, is the only paid member (the rest are volunteers). (REF. 18, p. 187)

717. (D) The Executive Board is the management body of the association. (REF. 23, p. 8)

718. (A) The AOTA national office is responsible for implementing association policies under the direction of the Executive Board. (REF. 23, p. 10)

719. (D) The executive director is appointed by the board as an employee of the association. (REF. 23, pp. 7-10)

720. (A) The executive director has, among other duties, management of the operations of the national office. (REF. 23, pp. 7-10)

721. (D) The WFOT is a formal organization apart from, but similar to, AOTA in that it has its own membership categories, committees, meetings, and delegates. (REF. 23, p. 9)

722. (C) The benefits offered to AOTA members are also available to the public. Some benefits are part of the membership "package" and some have additional costs or loan fees. People who

Management/Administration / 233

have paid for certification only can receive some of the same benefits free or at cost. (REF. 23, pp. 3-6)

723. (B) AOTA requires that a person pay separate fees for membership, for certification, and for the certification examination. (REF. 23, p. 3)

724. (B) The Award of Merit is the highest honor given by the AOTA. (REF. 9, p. B-19)

725. (D) The Eleanor Clarke Slagle Lectureship is the highest academic honor given by the AOTA. (REF. 9, p. B-21)

726. (A) An OTR is listed on the Roster of Fellows for a significant contribution. (REF. 9, p. B-23)

727. (C) A COTA is listed on the Roster of Honors for a significant contribution. (REF. 9, p. B-27)

728. (B) The AOTA has developed bylaws only for its own governance. (REF. 9, p. E-1)

729. (A) A member in good standing is one who has paid fees, agreed to uphold the standards and ethics of the association, and met the qualifications for membership. (REF. 9, p. E-1)

730. (B) The AOTA has developed two different sets of essentials: "Essentials of an Accredited Educational Program for the Occupational Therapist" and "Essentials of an Approved Program for the Occupational Therapy Assistant." (REF. 9, p. F-1)

731. (B) The AOTA has developed two different sets of examinations: "Certification Examination for Occupational Therapists, Registered" and "Certification Examination for Occupational Therapy Assistants." (REF. 18, p. 188)

732. (C) Puerto Rico has had a licensure law in effect since 1971, the earliest law for occupational therapists. (REF. 9, p. F-6)

733. (C) Indirect costs are usually delegated by square footage and are approximately 40% of the total budget. (REF. 15, p. 817)

734. (C) The formula for calculation of indirect costs of 40% for a $130,400 direct cost is

$$\frac{\text{Direct costs}}{X} = \frac{60\%}{40\%}$$

$$\frac{130,400}{X} = \frac{60\%}{40\%}$$

$$X = \frac{40\,(130,400)}{60}$$

$$X = 86,933$$

(REF. 15, p. 817)

735. (C) To determine total budget requirements, one must consider the direct costs, indirect costs, and bad debt allowance. (REF. 15, p. 817)

736. (B) To determine a fee for service, one must divide the total budget by the number of procedures projected for the budget period. (REF. 15, p. 817)

737. (B) To plan for a controlled budget, one must divide the total budget for the budget period by the number of projected budget procedures and by the number of months in the budget period, record the figures, and monitor the results for each unit of the budget period. (REF. 15, p. 817)

738. (C) To have a report understood at all levels, it must be written in a style acceptable within the facility's system. (REF. 15, p. 818)

739. (A) Research in occupational therapy is in its infancy. (REF. 15, p. 870)

740. (B) Much of the research that has been done in occupational therapy is descriptive of client characteristics or characteristics of occupational therapy or is concerned with occupational therapy education. (REF. 15, p. 872)

741. (B) Within the medical community the terms "referral" and "prescription" often are used interchangeably. (REF. 18, p. 146)

742. (D) A referral is the act of directing someone to a source for help; a prescription is a written instruction. Actual facts suggest that, in daily practice, both are significant. (REF. 18, p. 146)

743. (A) Most physicians are not knowledgeable enough about occupational therapy services to evaluate a person and select goals for therapy without input from an OTR. (REF. 18, p. 146)

744. (D) The fact remains that physicians are not trained in the use of many allied health professions, especially rehabilitation services. Thus the OTR needs to educate the physician about occupational therapy. (REF. 18, p. 146)

745. (A) If a physician knows a lot about occupational therapy services, then his/her role becomes one of coordination and management of the patient's services and details of implementation are left to the OTR. (REF. 18, p. 146)

746. (A) Occupational therapists may receive referrals from persons other than physicians, even from other agencies outside their own facility. (REF. 18, p. 147)

747. (C) Evaluation of a referral from a source other than a physician includes determination of the type of service needed in addition to occupational therapy or instead of occupational therapy, including the need for medical management and referral of the person to a physician if needed. (REF. 18, p. 147)

748. (A) If the referral is primarily for the purposes of developing a health maintenance or prevention program, a physician's consent may not be necessary. If a patient is under a physician's care or third-party payment is necessary, a consent is needed. (REF. 18, p. 147)

749. (C) Occupational therapists may refer individuals to other agencies, facilities, or professionals when services offered by these sources can be of benefit, or the OTR can refer indirectly by providing information to the individual for self-referral. (REF. 18, p. 147)

750. (B) The problem with blanket referrals is that some physicians never become aware of the goals or objectives established by the OTR for a specific person. (REF. 18, p. 147)

751. (D) OTRs must be alert to discourage the use of blanket referrals as a device to promote the use of occupational therapy as a diversional or recreational program. (REF. 18, p. 148)

752. (D) AOTA by a recent change in bylaws created the American Occupational Therapy Certification Board. This board has developed certification policies, procedures, and standard operating procedures for the certification of all OTRs and COTAs. (REF. 25, p. 1)

753. (B) The range of problems facing a manager is so great that one habitual set of responses or alternatives is inadequate. A manager must be able to perceive differences and tailor his/her style of action to fit the situation. Managers have no control of the range of problems that come their way. (REF. 26, p. 142)

754. (B) OTRs are responsible for participating in continuing education to ensure professional competence. No university program can teach new therapists all they need to know to practice. (REF. 18, p. 166)

755. (A) To keep up on new information OTRs need continuing education. Information is increasing and constantly changing and being revised. (REF. 18, p. 166)

756. (A) Quality assurance, according to the most recent Joint Commission on Accreditation of Hospitals policy statement, is concern with monitoring and evaluating the quality and appropriateness of patient care—not with discrimination, credentialing, licensure, or what has happened in patient care, but rather with making a particular thing happen. (REF. 26, pp. 253-257)

Management/Administration / 237

757. (C) Studies have shown that successful managers use participative management. This approach is complex but effective. The skill of building consensus is needed and the staff must come to a consensus on what the real problems are and how they will solve them. Managers must be active listeners, encourage expression of different views, deal with conflicts openly and candidly, and accept a solution that may differ from their own. (REF. 26, pp. 144-145)

758. (D) The primary difference between certification and licensure is that certification is granted by a nongovernmental agency or association, whereas licensure is granted by a governmental agency. (REF. 18, p. 149)

759. (A) Carefully kept records document the cause of intervention. (REF. 18, p. 160)

760. (C) In most cases the format of the records to be kept is outlined by regulations such as laws or policies in and for the institution. (REF. 18, p. 160)

761. (D) All records should include objective facts, augmented but not replaced by subjective feelings that should be based upon objective facts. (REF. 18, p. 160)

762. (A) In record keeping, facts that can be measured should be used to the maximum extent possible. (REF. 18, p. 160)

763. (A) Prevention of further injury or illness involves all of the safety factors known and knowledge about a person's progress in a specific in a specific disorder. The therapist must take whatever action is necessary to prevent further injury or illness by calling it to the attention of the family, the person who has the problem, and other team members. (REF. 18, p. 154)

764. (B) General Systems Theory is a theoretical model. The main objective of a general systems approach is to develop a framework for communication between specialists to allow the entire system to function and meet objectives in a complex environment like today's health care system. (REF. 15, p. 799)

765. (C) General Systems Theory has no specific methodology. It accepts the complexities of the system and searches for the structural patterns that will enable one to examine the problem as a whole. (REF. 15, p. 799)

766. (A) The problem with the systems approach is that it lacks clarity. Its framework is built on communication, which breaks down, there is a constant need for arbitration of conflicts between various members of the agency, and it demands absolute clarity of objectives. Objectives for each individual must be derived from the objectives as a whole. (REF. 15, p. 800)

767. (B) The skill gained from a systems approach assists the occupational therapy manager and individual clinician in gaining power. Sometimes the person in authority is not the one with power. (REF. 15, p. 813)

768. (B) A manager with power has more opportunity to be creative and to explore, while a manager without power has no choice but to maintain control over activities within his/her own jurisdiction. Authority is defined as the right to give commands; power is influence built through positive, carefully planned means. (REF. 15, p. 813)

769. (D) The budget is a management tool. Through it the occupational therapy manager/director has the ability to establish programs by obtaining financial support. (REF. 15, p. 816)

770. (A) Staff functions require that both the quality and/or the number of persons necessary to accomplish the objectives be identified. (REF. 15, p. 819)

771. (B) In the hiring of an occupational therapist to fill a job, a job specification form is prepared on the basis of the job description. The job specification identifies the minimum acceptable qualifications for the specific position, including experience, education, and other data. (REF. 15, p. 820)

772. (C) The Privacy Act of 1974 limits information that can be obtained to that which verifies actual employment in a certain job for a certain time period at a certain level of compensation. (REF. 15, p. 822)

773. (C) During the interview process, it is important to discuss the actual job requirements to see if the applicant is qualified, but it is also important to determine if the applicant's job expectations can be met in the particular position. (REF. 15, p. 822)

774. (B) During the induction phase it is the employee's responsibility to develop interpersonal skills and acquire additional knowledge about the job and the history of the organization. However, if proper attention has been given to the organization's recruitment, interviews, and the completion of an induction program, the new employee should be able to perform all the job functions required in the job description. (REF. 15, p. 822)

775. (C) The primary purpose of a person's medical records is to document the person's course of health care. Use of the record for other than direct patient care requires the person's authorization; however, a record may be subpoenaed by the courts without the person's consent. (REF. 15, p. 823)

776. (D) The medical records department of a facility is responsible for designing and implementing the record-keeping system. (REF. 15, p. 823)

777. (B) The Medical Records, Medical Evaluations, and Patient Case, developed by Laurence Weld, M.D., constitutes the "weed system," which is the "problem-oriented" medical record better known as the SOAP system. (REF. 15, p. 820)

778. (A) The purpose of a code of ethics for health care providers is to describe the relationships among the client, the practitioners, and the public or society. (REF. 18, p. 160)

779. (B) AOTA has established the Principles of Occupational Therapy Ethics intended for all occupational therapy personnel. Most ethical standards are supported by law in some form. If a person can prove she/he was damaged by unethical practice, the person may initiate a civil suit and, if successful, may collect damages

as compensation. Therefore, ethics should not be considered separately from the law. (REF. 26, p. 360)

780. (C) AOTA's Principles of Occupational Therapy Ethics were intended to be action-oriented, guiding, and preventive rather than negative or merely disciplinary and were not intended as a definition of standards for health care. (REF. 18, p. 261)

781. (D) The Principles of Occupational Therapy Ethics were established by AOTA for internal use only. (REF. 18, p. 261)

782. (D) The code of ethics of AOTA states that a therapist in dealing with other professionals shall take action according to established procedures when he/she has objective evidence of a breach of ethics or substandard service. (REF. 18, p. 262)

783. (A) Strategic planning is a necessary part of health care planning. When health care providers fail to offer services that address society's needs and purposes at any time the organization may lose its edge in the marketplace and take on the probability of failure. (REF. 15, p. 839)

784. (C) If the occupational therapy manager does not have access to the developmental portion of a strategic plan he/she will be able to do little more than react to changes, and decisions regarding the department will be little more than arbitrary. (REF. 15, p. 838)

785. (A) In reviewing each service with respect to its relevance to society's purposes and organizational goals, if a service would not be reconsidered it would be dropped from the department's plan for future use. (REF. 15, p. 840)

786. (C) Quality assurance is best described by the assessment of actual service delivery and its health care outcomes. (REF. 15, p. 861)

787. (B) It has been said that theories consist of statements that relate concepts. Concepts are ways of classifying the world around us. In research about occupational therapy, concepts are often either unclearly defined or not defined at all and it is extremely difficult to agree upon the meaning of the concepts. Occupational therapy thus far has few concepts that have operational definitions. (REF. 15, p. 870)

788. (A) In occupational therapy today, very few theories exist that allow knowledge to be developed and tested. Little confidence can be held in the theories that do exist since very few data support the statements constituting the theories in occupational therapy. (REF. 15, p. 870)

789. (B) Occupational therapy practice, for the most part, is based upon tradition and untested hypotheses. (REF. 15, p. 870)

790. (A) In two surveys of the *American Journal of Occupational Therapy*, in 1973 and 1979, the quantity and type of research papers remained approximately the same; 44% of the papers published were research papers. (REF. 15, p. 871)

791. (C) Much of the research that has been done in occupational therapy so far is descriptive of client characteristics and occupational therapist characteristics or is concerned with the outcomes of occupational therapy education. (REF. 15, p. 872)

792. (D) Occupational therapy's current state of research represents a stage in the normal evolution of professional knowledge, which proceeds from the intuitive practice of an untested art to the logically rigorous practice of a science. (REF. 15, p. 872)

793. (C) Role assignments to a department or a given staff must always be based on the discipline's and/or individual staff's professional preparation to provide a service. Role definitions cannot routinely be made on the basis of modalities used but should be based on why and how a modality is used. (REF. 24, p. 7)

794. (A) Staffing pattern and staff ratios will depend on the nature of the patient population. Budgets must be developed to meet these ratios. (REF. 24, p. 17)

795. (B) Ideally, nonsupervisory staff should spend 60% of their time in direct patient care and approximately 40% in support services. These percentages will depend on many factors: the

manager, the supervisor, the center, and the need for patient services. (REF. 24, p. 17)

796. (C) A psychiatric occupational therapy staff-to-patient ratio of 1 to 22 is suggested. (REF. 24, p. 17)

797. (B) In the staffing pattern the ratio of two assistants to each professional occupational therapist should not be exceeded. If COTAs are not available, then a ratio of one aide to one OTR would apply. (REF. 25, p. 17)

798. (B) There is continuous debate about the relative merits of a decentralized hospital structure as compared with a centralized model. Administrative staff most frequently support a decentralized system with relatively autonomous sections. (REF. 24, p. 19)

799. (A) Professional services staff usually favor a centralized model with relatively autonomous departments accountable to a professional department head who is generally responsible to a clinical director. (REF. 24, p. 19)

800. (D) Too often a manager in planning development or redirecting a program addresses what changes must be made rather than what the program model should look like in the future. (REF. 24, p. 45)

References

1. Williams, P. L., and Warwick, R. (Eds.): *Gray's Anatomy,* 36th ed. W. B. Saunders, Philadelphia, 1980.

2. Hollinshead, W., and Jenkins, B.: *Functional Anatomy of the Limbs and Back,* 5th ed. W. B. Saunders, Philadelphia, 1981.

3. Quiring, D. P., and Warfel, J. H. (Eds.): *The Extremities,* 5th ed. Lea and Febiger, Philadelphia, 1985.

4. Wells, F., and Luttgens, K.: *Kinesiology,* 7th ed. W. B. Saunders, Philadelphia, 1982.

5. Guyton, A.: *Physiology of the Human Body,* 6th ed. W. B. Saunders, Philadelphia, 1984.

6. Schottelius, B. A., and Schottleius, D. C.: *Textbook of Physiology,* 18th ed. C. V. Mosby, St. Louis, 1978.

7. Chusid, J. G., and McDonald, J. J.: *Correlative Neuroanatomy and Functional Neurology,* 19th ed. Lange Medical Publications, Los Altos, CA, 1985.

8. Everett, N. B.: *Functional Neuroanatomy,* 6th ed. Lea and Febiger, Philadelphia, 1971.

9. *AOTA Member Handbook,* American Occupational Therapy Association, Rockville, MD, 1980.

10. Cynkin, S.: *Occupational Therapy: Toward Health Through Activities,* Little, Brown, Boston, 1979.

11. Kolb, L. C.: *Modern Clinical Psychiatry,* 10th ed. W. B. Saunders, Philadelphia, 1982.

12. Boyd, W., and Huntington, S.: *Introduction to the Study of Disease,* 9th ed. Lea and Febiger, Philadelphia, 1984.

13. Rusk, H. A.: *Rehabilitation Medicine,* 4th ed. C. V. Mosby, St. Louis, 1977.

14. Taber, C. W.: *Taber's Cyclopedic Medical Dictionary,* 15th ed. F. A. Davis, Philadelphia, 1985.

15. Hopkins, H. L., and Smith, H. D. (Eds.): *Willard and Spackman's Occuptional Therapy,* 6th ed. J. B. Lippincott, Philadelphia, 1983.

16. Trombly, C. A., and Scott, A. D.: *Occupational Therapy for Physical Dysfunction,* 2nd ed. Williams and Wilkins, Baltimore, 1983.

17. Banus, B. S., et al.: *The Developmental Therapist,* 2nd ed. Slack, Thorofare, NJ, 1979.

18. Reed, K., and Sanderson, S. R.: *Concepts of Occupational Therapy,* 2nd ed. Williams and Wilkins, Baltimore, 1983.

19. Lewis, S. C.: *The Mature Years: A Geriatric Occupational Therapy Text.* Slack, Thorofare, NJ, 1979.

20. Kielhofner, G. (Ed.): *A Model of Human Occupation: Theory and Application.* Williams and Wilkins, Baltimore, 1985.

21. Pedretti, L. W. (Ed.): *Occupational Therapy: Practice Skills for Physical Dysfunction,* 2nd ed. C. V. Mosby, St. Louis, 1985.

22. Reed, K. L.: *Models of Practice in Occupational Therapy.* Williams and Wilkins, Baltimore, 1984.

23. *AOTA Member Handbook*. American Occupational Therapy Association, Rockville, MD, 1984.

24. Fidler, G. S.: *Design of Rehabilitation Services in Psychiatric Hospital Settings*. Ramsco Publishing Co., Laurel, MD, 1984.

25. American Occupational Therapy Association: *Occupational Therapy News*, Vol. 41, No. 1, January 1987.

26. Blair, J., and Gray, M. (Eds.): *The Occupational Therapy Manager*. American Occupational Therapy Association, Rockville, MD, 1985.

27. Hemphill, B. J.: *The Evaluative Process in Psychiatric Occupational Therapy*. Slack, Thorofare, NJ, 1982.

28. Howe, M. C., and Schwartzberg, S. L.: *A Functional Approach to Group Work in Occupational Therapy*, J. B. Lippincott, New York, 1986.